Quick Guide to Anaphylaxis

Cemal Cingi • Nuray Bayar Muluk

Quick Guide
to Anaphylaxis

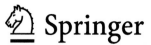 Springer

Cemal Cingi
ENT Department
Faculty of Medicine
Eskişehir Osmangazi
University
Eskisehir, Turkey

Nuray Bayar Muluk
ENT Department
Faculty of Medicine
Kırıkkale University
Kırıkkale, Turkey

ISBN 978-3-030-33638-7   ISBN 978-3-030-33639-4   (eBook)
DOI 10.1007/978-3-030-33639-4

This Springer imprint is published by the registered company Springer Nature Switzerland AG
The registered company address is: Gewerbestrasse 11, 6330 Cham, Switzerland

Preface

Anaphylaxis always puts me in mind of a thunderstorm far out at sea.

Managing anaphylaxis is rather like attempting to sail a boat safely through the eye of a raging storm. Just like the storm, anaphylaxis may appear suddenly and without warning, terrifying anyone caught up in it. Each step taken must be exactly correct, swift, timely and in the right order, despite the feeling of panic that surrounds such an occurrence. If this panic affects even seasoned health professionals faced with anaphylaxis, just imagine how much more deeply terrified it must make the patient and family members feel.

In this frenzied atmosphere, all of us need to stay calm and authoritative, bringing the patient calmly towards safety. The aim of this book is to give you a guidebook and a map to guide you through the choppy waters of anaphylaxis, so that you, too, can act as an expert helmsman to your patients caught up in the storm of anaphylaxis. I would like to add my sincere heartfelt thanks to my distinguished co-author, **Nuray Bayar Muluk**, for her unwavering enthusiasm, patience, and deep insights.

I hope that this book proves to be of great help to you.

Best wishes from

Eskisehir, Turkey   Cemal Cingi

Contents

About the Authors

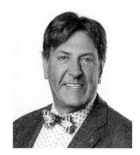

Cemal Cingi, MD, is a Professor in the Otorhinolaryngology Department at Eskisehir Osmangazi University, Medical Faculty, Eskisehir, Turkey. He graduated from the School of Medicine, Istanbul University, in 1984 and then entered the Otorhinolaryngology Residency Programme at Anadolu University, Eskisehir, becoming a Specialist in ORL and HNS in 1990. He was appointed as an Associate Professor in 1995 and as a Professor in 2001. In 2013, he became an accredited Specialist in Mouth, Face, and Chin Surgery. Dr. Cingi served as the Chair of the ENT Section of the European Academy of Allergy and Clinical Immunology (EAACI) and President of the Asian Facial Plastic Surgery Society (AFPSS). He is the editor of the journal *ENT Updates* and an editorial board member for several other journals.

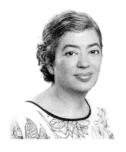

Nuray Bayar Muluk, MD, has been a Professor in the Otorhinolaryngology Department at Kirikkale University Faculty of Medicine, Turkey, since 2008. At present, she is the Head of the Department. She graduated from Hacettepe University Faculty of Medicine in 1990 and completed her ENT residency at the same University in 1994. Her interests include basic research, rhinology, and allergy. She has published 225 international and 70 national papers, and she is a co-editor of 2 international books, 6 national books, and 2 translated books. She has more than 75 book chapters. She is an associate editor of *ENT Updates.*

Chapter 1
Anaphylaxis: Definition, History, and Epidemiology

1.1 Definition of Anaphylaxis

Anaphylaxis can lead to death, but even so, rates of diagnosis
and levels of treatment remain low. In part, not understanding
that anaphylaxis covers more than simply "anaphylactic shock",
and that treating the disorder depends upon identifying the syndrome rapidly and stopping, by judicious use of epinephrine, the
potentially lethal cardiovascular and respiratory complications,
may be to blame [1].

Anaphylaxis lies at the severe end of a spectrum of acute
allergy responses which affect multiple body systems. In clinical
practice, anaphylactic signs are observed in several organs, usually beginning with skin signs before next involving the respiratory system, also reacting on the gut and producing cardiovascular
alteration, until the heart and breathing are arrested in the last
phase. Anaphylaxis, strictly speaking, refers to the immunological response working through IgE and, to a lesser extent, IgG and
IgM (Coombs and Gell Type 3 reactions). Anaphylactoid (pseudo-
allergic) is, by contrast, the term used in cases showing a similar
clinical profile but not attributable to antibody formation. Some
recent classification attempts have put such syndromes under the
anaphylactic label, extending usage to mean any acute reaction
involving hypersensitivity and affecting the whole body [2].

© Springer Nature Switzerland AG 2020   1
C. Cingi, N. B. Muluk, *Quick Guide to Anaphylaxis*,
https://doi.org/10.1007/978-3-030-33639-4_1

Anaphylaxis is definable as a life-threatening response, acute in onset, involving many organs and initiated by mast cell and basophilic degranulation [3, 4]. Archetypally, previous exposure to an allergen induces sensitivity, which, upon second exposure, incites an immunological response [5]. The main culprits are allergens in food, implicated in 33–56% of incidences overall and approaching 81% in paediatric cases [6–8].

The principal systems with involvement in anaphylaxis are the skin, gut, respiratory, and cardiovascular systems. Fully developed anaphylaxis features urticarial, angioedematous (with consequent hypotension), and bronchospastic responses [5]. However, no one clinical definition is agreed upon by all authorities. Clinicians rely on the habitual systemic features and, frequently, documented exposure to an antigenic stimulus, to make the diagnosis [5].

Laboratory confirmation is seldom necessary or beneficial in what is, in essence, a purely clinical diagnosis. In case of unclarity, particularly where a chronic element is present, or other conditions need to be considered, the laboratory may be of some limited assistance in the provision of IgE serology, as may dermal prick tests [5]. Immediate action to recognise and treat anaphylaxis is essential—it is an emergency, but the actual treatment varies according to the initial severity and how the patient responds clinically to intervention [5].

Whilst anaphylaxis is most frequently attributable to medications, food or additives, other sources of allergens as well as non-chemical initiators (temperature extremes or ultraviolet irradiation) exist. How anaphylaxis unfolds clinically and how severely, hinges upon both the level to which the patient is sensitised and other elements present at the time of exposure: infection, physical exercise, emotional pressure, and other medicinal drug use, such as beta adrenoceptor antagonists. A high percentage of otherwise unexplained (idiopathic) anaphylactic reactions may conceivably be due to this "summation anaphylaxis". Cases due to insect stings have levels of angiotensin in blood that are inversely correlated with the degree of reaction, a severe reaction showing lower angiotensin and vice versa [2].

1.2 History

Anaphylaxis as a term dates to Portier and Richet's study in 1902 in which a dog died as a result of receiving two consecutive doses of sea anemone toxin, the second after a delay. It is made up of the Greek terms *ana-* (again, up) and *-phylaxis* (protection, immunity) [5].

Paul Portier and Charles Richet did the key study, but in fact, Megendie had also noted that a substance which one would not normally expect to be lethal could cause a generalised reaction ending in death. He injected egg albumin sequentially into rabbits, which suddenly collapsed and died [9]. For the following few decades, researchers observed that laboratory animals could have a life-threatening reaction to non-self-materials, even when at levels that previously caused no apparent problem. Richet, in concert with Portier, isolated the toxin found in tentacles of the genus *Physalia* (the Portuguese man-of-war) as well as the venom of the *Actinia sulcata*, an anemone found in prolific numbers at the French seaside, and closely related to the *Physalia* toxin. They were attempting to establish what constituted a lethal dosage of the toxin in dogs, and, assuming that those animals who survived being given a first dose would now carry immunity to the toxin, they were astonished instead to discover that lower levels of the toxin given subsequently were in fact lethal in a short space of time [10]. In explaining the finding as an apparent lack of immunity following innoculation with toxin, Richet coined the term "aphylaxis", subsequently settling on "anaphylaxis" as a more euphonious combination of letters [11]. But, even though the terminology dates to over a century ago, defining the actual phenomenon it denotes in a consistent way has been less straightforward [12].

Anaphylaxis is archetypally a severe reaction, affecting skin, gut, lungs, and heart [13]. Generally, such a picture is readily identified by doctors, but the presence of few or less severe symptoms can complicate diagnosis. An "immediate systemic reaction caused by rapid, IgE [immunoglobulin E]-mediated immune release of potent mediators from tissue mast cells and peripheral basophils" is how the 1998 Joint Task Force of the American Academy of Allergy, Asthma and Immunology (AAAAI) and the American College of Allergy, Asthma and Immunology (ACAAI) describe an anaphylactic reaction [14]. However, since some reactions can "mimic signs and symptoms of anaphylaxis but are caused by non-IgE-mediated release of potent mediators from mast cells and basophils", they are described as "anaphylactoid" rather than "anaphylactic", a complicated situation for the clinician working in a clinic or Accident and Emergency, who may recognise the syndrome but be unaware of the underlying mechanism, which the above scheme bases the distinction upon. The definition of anaphylaxis as "a serious allergic reaction that is rapid in onset and may cause death" [15] emerged from two later symposia. Criteria to diagnose anaphylaxis in clinical settings were outlined by the Second Symposium on the Definition and Management of Anaphylaxis [12, 15].

1.3 Epidemiology of Anaphylaxis

It is unknown what the actual incidence of all-cause anaphylaxis in the general population is [16–18]. Estimates based upon occurrence in communities are complicated by low rates of diagnosis and incomplete documentation, coupled with erroneous coding practice, concomitant use of differing case definitions, and ways to quantify the incidence [18–20]. Nonetheless, anaphylaxis is evidently not a seldom-seen phenomenon and incidence is on the rise, particularly in childhood and early adulthood [21–23].

Anaphylaxis occurs 30 times in every 100,000 person-years [24, 25], with the most severe forms put at the level of 5–15 per 100,000 [26]. Using data gathered routinely when admitting patients to hospital in the UK, some studies recorded a 700% increase in anaphylactic incidence between 1990/1 and 2003/4, noting the incidence to be highest in children of school age [27, 28]. Quantification of paediatric risk of anaphylaxis is hampered by a paucity of relevant data. Since different ways were used for defining anaphylaxis in the data that are available, this presents methodological issues to researchers. To illustrate the problem, whilst incidence in children equals that of adults in some studies [29, 30], elsewhere it is quoted as a mere 0.19 in 100,000 [31], although this figure is likely to be on the low side due to the method used to calculate it [32]. A variety of techniques have been employed to reveal the epidemiological aspects of anaphylaxis. One study looking at all school students in France gauged that 1 in 1000 had a plan to manage their anaphylaxis. The increasing rate of epinephrine prescription mirrors the increase in awareness of risks attributable to allergies: in the UK, children born between 1990 and 1992 were seven times more likely to have an Epipen than those born 9 years earlier [33]; in Canada, 1% of the population is in possession of a prescription for epinephrine, rising to 5% in boys between 1 year and 17 months old [34].

Anaphylaxis incidence is on the rise, especially in patients up to the age of 20, most frequently triggered by foodstuffs, medicinal drugs, or insect venom. To make the diagnosis, a careful history establishing that the patient has been exposed to the putative offending agent, with a typical symptomatic and clinical pattern ensuing, needs to be recorded. On occasion, serum tryptase elevation may be indicative. It is worth investigating atypical presentations of anaphylaxis as a way of identifying unsuspected causes and ways for anaphylaxis to develop. Cases determined to be idiopathic on account of negative dermal tests and IgE serology may be due to an unsuspected allergen or may be a manifestation of mastocytosis or clonal mast cell disorder, so these possibilities must be entertained [35].

The variety of criteria used in the diagnosis of anaphylaxis ensures that the actual incidence of the disorder continues to be unknown. Hospital—or health maintenance organization—(HMO)-based studies have given results ranging between 30–60 cases per 100,000 and 2000 events per 100,000, equating to 0.03–2.0% risk of developing the disease in a lifetime [36]. Anaphylaxis may in fact still be underreported due to the diagnosis of allergic reaction being used where several physiological systems are involved, in place of the more precise anaphylaxis descriptor [20]. An audit of case notes for Accident and Emergency revealed that in 678 cases, anaphylaxis had been wrongly classified as food allergy. Another research team found that 617 cases in which an insect had stung the patient and which reached the threshold for a diagnosis for anaphylaxis had not been so diagnosed [37, 38]. The reasons why neither victims nor clinicians consider the anaphylaxis diagnosis may be multifactorial. Where episodes are unique and repetition in symptomatology is not observed, the involvement of IgE may be overlooked. Although the majority of anaphylactic reactions triggered by food happen in minutes from the exposure, meat of mammalian animals may not trigger a reaction for a number of hours post ingestion [39]. If the victim is a small child or one with communication problems arising from disease, neither the patient nor carer may realise what has happened. Symptoms may be masked by drugs used for other conditions, such as classical H_1 antagonists. If clinicians do not take a full history and examine the patient carefully, anaphylaxis will pass unnoticed, and even where this is undertaken, if urticaria or other dermal signs are not present, the clinician may miss the diagnosis [16, 20].

A cohort study made feasible by the Rochester Epidemiology Project and conducted retrospectively revealed doubling of anaphylactic incidence between the 1980s and 1990s (21 in 100,000 to 49.8 in 100,000) [21]. The peak incidence was situated in those under the age of 19 (70 in 100,000). Comparable results have emerged from other research [22, 23]. Up to their 15th year, boys are more likely to be affected than girls, but this pattern then reverses after age 15. The most common trigger in children, adolescents, and younger adults is food, but in midlife and beyond, drug treatments and insects assume greater significance, alongside unknown causes [17].

Anaphylaxis seldom results in death, it seems [40–44], but this may be an artefact, since missing clinical details, not performing a careful search of the surrounding area where a death has occurred, non-specific post-mortem results, the non-existence of perfectly specific and sensitive diagnostic pathological tests and a tendency to misclassify the condition all probably contribute to a falsely low incidence [19, 20].

A clinical audit in the west of the USA undertaken in a big healthcare provider discovered that 35% of cases labelled anaphylactic shock (ICD9-CM 995.0) as well as 87.3% anaphylactic shock secondary to adverse food reaction (ICD9-CM 995.3) lacked supporting clinical details for anaphylaxis to be confidently diagnosed [45]. If no signs are present, a symptomatic history only (e.g. abdominodynia or pruritus) may not alert the clinician to anaphylaxis. Since there is symptomatic overlap with other conditions, the history needs to be precisely taken to be sure it represents anaphylaxis and not factitious disorder imposed on self or another, or seafood poisoning [20]. In spite of the limitations on the data arising from lack of recognition or confounding with other disorders, it can be demonstrated that there has been a significant rise in anaphylaxis episodes [12, 21, 22, 27, 46–48].

Children who suffer anaphylaxis usually have the reaction triggered by food allergies [49–51]. A study which looked back over 3 years' worth of children's Accident and Emergency records in Australia showed three main causes of anaphylaxis: food, medication, and insect venom (56%, 5%, and 5%, respectively), with the remaining cases lacking a documented trigger [30]. The medications most frequently cited as cause to the Allergy Vigilance Network are anti-microbials, especially penicillin-class and β-lactams [26]. Severe anaphylaxis occurring under anaesthesia is still most often attributable to muscle relaxants [52, 53]. Paediatric patients with known allergic problems, spina bifida, or having repeat surgery are especially prone to anaphylaxis triggered by latex [54, 55]. Specific immunotherapy is also known to trigger anaphylaxis [56]. Finally, there are reactions which do not fit into the above schema and are therefore termed idiopathic. The paediatric incidence is unknown [57].

Severe anaphylaxis has an associated mortality of 0.65–2% [6, 58], translating to 1–3 deaths annually per million population. An American review of 32 deaths caused by anaphylaxis triggered by allergy to food [50] found an age range of 2–33 years, acute severe spasm of the bronchi having happened in the majority (96%) of these. Similar figures have emerged from the UK [59]. Of the 32 US deaths, 63% were caused by peanut, whilst other nuts from trees explained a further 31%. The remainder were attributed to dairy products or fish. It is calculated that anaphylaxis triggered by food claims 150 lives every year in the USA [50].

References

1. Campbell RL, Kelso JM. Anaphylaxis: emergency treatment. In: Walls RM, Randolph AG. Feldweg AM, editors. UpToDate. Last updated: Jun 07, 2016. http://www.uptodate.com/contents/anaphylaxis-emergency-treatment. Accessed online at 24 June 2016.
2. Ring J, Brockow K, Behrendt H. History and classification of anaphylaxis. Novartis Found Symp. 2004;257:6–16; discussion 16–24, 45–50, 276–85.
3. Kemp SF, Lockey RF. Anaphylaxis: a review of causes and mechanisms. J Allergy Clin Immunol. 2002;110(3):341–8.
4. Simons FE, Anaphylaxis J. Allergy Clin Immunol. 2008;121(2 Suppl):S402–7; quiz S420.
5. Mustafa SS. Anaphylaxis. In: Kaliner MA, editor. Medscape. http://emedicine.medscape.com/article/135065-overview#showall. Accessed online at 24 June 2016.
6. Ben-Shoshan M, Clarke AE. Anaphylaxis: past, present and future. Allergy. 2011;66:1–14.
7. Cianferoni A, Novembre E, Mugnaini L, Lombardi E, Bernardini R, Pucci N, et al. Clinical features of acute anaphylaxis in patients admitted to a university hospital: an 11-year retrospective review (1985-1996). Ann Allergy Asthma Immunol. 2001;87:27–32.
8. Wang J, Sampson HA. Food anaphylaxis. Clin Exp Allergy. 2007;37:651–60.
9. Megendie F. Lectures on blood. Philadelphia: Aswell, Barrington and Haswell; 1839.
10. Cohen SG, Mazzullo JC. Discovering anaphylaxis: elucidation of a shocking phenomenon. J Allergy Clin Immunol. 2009;124:866–869. e1.
11. May CD. The ancestry of allergy: being an account of the original experimental induction of hypersensitivity recognizing the contribution of Paul Portier. J Allergy Clin Immunol. 1985;75:485–95.

12. Boden SR, Burks AW. Anaphylaxis: a history with emphasis on food allergy. Immunol Rev. 2011;242(1):247–57.
13. Sampson HA, et al. Symposium on the definition and management of anaphylaxis: summary report. J Allergy Clin Immunol. 2005;115:584–91.
14. Joint Task Force on Practice Parameters, American Academy of Allergy, Asthma and Immunology, American College of Allergy, Asthma and Immunology, and the Joint Council of Allergy, Asthma and Immunology. The diagnosis and management of anaphylaxis. J Allergy Clin Immunol. 1998;101:S465–528.
15. Sampson HA, Muñoz-Furlong A, Campbell RL, Adkinson NF Jr, Bock SA, Branum A, et al. Second symposium on the definition and management of anaphylaxis: summary report—Second National Institute of Allergy and Infectious Disease/Food Allergy and Anaphylaxis Network symposium. J Allergy Clin Immunol. 2006;117(2):391–7.
16. Tejedor-Alonso MA, Moro-Moro M, Múgica-García MV. Epidemiology of anaphylaxis: contributions from the last 10 years. J Investig Allergol Clin Immunol. 2015;25(3):163–75; quiz follow 174–5. Review.
17. Lieberman PL. Anaphylaxis. In: Adkinson Jr NF, Bochner BS, Busse WW, Holgate ST, Lemanske Jr RF, Simons FER, editors. Middleton's allergy: principles and practice. 7th ed. St Louis: Mosby, Inc; 2009. p. 1027–49.
18. Clark S, Camargo CA Jr. Epidemiology of anaphylaxis. Immunol Allergy Clin N Am. 2007;27(2):145–63.
19. Clark S, Gaeta TJ, Kamarthi GS, Camargo CA. ICD-9-CM coding of emergency department visits for food and insect sting allergy. Ann Epidemiol. 2006;16(9):696–700. Epub 2006 Mar 3.
20. Simons FER, Sampson HA. Anaphylaxis epidemic: fact or fiction? J Allergy Clin Immunol. 2008;122:1166–8.
21. Decker WW, Campbell RL, Manivannan V, Luke A, St Sauver JL, Weaver A, et al. The etiology and incidence of anaphylaxis in Rochester, Minnesota: a report from the Rochester Epidemiology Project. J Allergy Clin Immunol. 2008;122(6):1161–5.
22. Lin RY, Anderson AS, Shah SN, Nurruzzaman F. Increasing anaphylaxis hospitalizations in the first 2 decades of life: New York State, 1990-2006. Ann Allergy Asthma Immunol. 2008;101: 387–93.
23. Sheikh A, Hippisley-Cox J, Newton J, Fenty J. Trends in national incidence, lifetime prevalence and adrenaline prescribing for anaphylaxis in England. J R Soc Med. 2008;101(3):139–43. https://doi.org/10.1258/jrsm.2008.070306.

24. Muraro A, Roberts G, Clark A, Eigenmann PA, Halken S, Lack G, Moneret-Vautrin A, Niggemann B, Rancé F. EAACI Task Force on Anaphylaxis in Children. The management of anaphylaxis in childhood: position paper of the European Academy of Allergology and Clinical Immunology. Allergy. 2007;62(8):857–71. Epub 2007 Jun 21

25. Yocum MW, Butterfield JH, Klein JS, Volcheck GW, Schroeder DR, Silverstein MD. Epidemiology of anaphylaxis in Olmsted Country: a population-based study. J Allergy Clin Immunol. 1999;104:452–6.

26. Moneret-Vautrin DA, Morisset M, Flabbee J, Beaudouin E, Kanny G. Epidemiology of life-threatening and lethal anaphylaxis: a review. Allergy. 2005;60:443–51.

27. Sheikh A, Alves B. Hospital admissions for acute anaphylaxis: time trend study. BMJ. 2000;320:1441.

28. Gupta R, Sheikh A, Strachan DP, Anderson HR. Time trends in allergic disorders in the UK. Thorax. 2007;62:91–6.

29. Bohlke K, Davis RL, De Stefano F, Mary SM, Braun MM, Thompson RS. Epidemiology of anaphylaxis among children and adolescents enrolled in a health maintenance organization. J Allergy Clin Immunol. 2004;113:536–42.

30. Braganza SC, Acworth JP, Mckinnon DR, Peake JE, Brown AF. Paediatric emergency department anaphylaxis: different patterns from adults. Arch Dis Child. 2006;91:159–63.

31. Macdougall CF, Cant AJ, Colver AF. How dangerous is food allergy in childhood? The incidence of severe and fatal allergic reactions across the UK and Ireland. Arch Dis Child. 2002;86:236–9.

32. Clark AT, Ewan PW. Food allergy in childhood. Arch Dis Child. 2004;89:197.

33. Morritt J, Aszkenasy M. The anaphylaxis problem in children: community management in a UK National Health Service district. Public Health. 2000;14:456–9.

34. Simons F, Peterson S, Black CD. Epinephrine dispensing patterns for an out of-hospital population: a novel approach to studying the epidemiology of anaphylaxis. J Allergy Clin Immunol. 2002;110:647–51.

35. Simons FE. Anaphylaxis: recent advances in assessment and treatment. J Allergy Clin Immunol. 2009;124(4):625–36.; ; quiz 637–8. https://doi.org/10.1016/j.jaci.2009.08.025.

36. Lieberman P, Camargo CA Jr, Bohlke K, Jick H, Miller RL, Sheikh A, Simons FE. Epidemiology of anaphylaxis: findings of the American College of Allergy, Asthma and Immunology Epidemiology of Anaphylaxis Working Group. Ann Allergy Asthma Immunol. 2006;97:596–602.

37. Gaeta TJ, Clark S, Pelletier AJ, Camargo CA. National study of US emergency department visits for acute allergic reactions, 1993 to 2004. Ann Allergy Asthma Immunol. 2007;98:360–5.
38. Clark S, Long AA, Gaeta TJ, Camargo CA Jr. Multicenter study of emergency department visits for insect sting allergies. J Allergy Clin Immunol. 2005;116:643–9.
39. Commins SP, Satinover SM, Hosen J, Mozena J, Borish L, Lewis BD, et al. Delayed anaphylaxis, angioedema, or urticaria after consumption of red meat in patients with IgE antibodies specific for galactose-alpha-1,3-galactose. J Allergy Clin Immunol. 2009;123:426–33.
40. Sampson HA, Mendelson L, Rosen JP. Fatal and near-fatal anaphylactic reactions to food in children and adolescents. N Engl J Med. 1992;327(6):380–4.
41. Bock SA, Muñoz-Furlong A, Sampson HA. Further fatalities caused by anaphylactic reactions to food, 2001-2006. J Allergy Clin Immunol. 2007;119(4):1016–8. Epub 2007 Feb 15.
42. Pumphrey RS, Gowland MH. Further fatal allergic reactions to food in the United Kingdom, 1999-2006. J Allergy Clin Immunol. 2007;119(4):1018–9.. Epub 2007 Mar 8.
43. Greenberger PA, Rotskoff BD, Lifschultz B. Fatal anaphylaxis: postmortem findings and associated comorbid diseases. Ann Allergy Asthma Immunol. 2007;98(3):252–7.
44. Liew WK, Williamson E, Tang ML. Anaphylaxis fatalities and admissions in Australia. J Allergy Clin Immunol. 2009;123(2):434–42. https://doi.org/10.1016/j.jaci.2008.10.049. Epub 2008 Dec 30.
45. Bohlke K, Davis RL, DeStefano F, Marcy SM, Braun MM, Thompson RS, et al. Epidemiology of anaphylaxis among children and adolescents enrolled in a health maintenance organization. J Allergy Clin Immunol. 2004;113(3):536–42.
46. Gupta R, et al. Time trends in allergic disorders in the UK. Thorax. 2007;62:91–6.
47. Poulos LM, Waters AM, Correll PK, Loblay RH, Marks GB. Trends in hospitalizations for anaphylaxis, angioedema, and urticaria in Australia, 1993–1994 to 2004–2005. J Allergy Clin Immunol. 2007;120(4):878–84.
48. Simon MR, Mulla BD. A population-based epidemiologic analysis of deaths from anaphylaxis in Florida. Allergy. 2008;63:1077–83.
49. Novembre E, Cianferoni A, Bernardini R, Mugnaini L, Caffarelli C, Cavagni G, et al. Anaphylaxis in children: clinical and allergologic features. Pediatrics. 1998;101:8–16.
50. Bock SA, Munoz-Furlong A, Sampson HA. Fatalities dues to anaphylactic reactions to foods. J Allergy Clin Immunol. 2001;107:191–3.

51. Mehl A, Wahn U, Niggemann B. Anaphylactic reactions in children—a questionnaire based survey in Germany. Allergy. 2005;60:1440 5.
52. Mertes PM, Laxenaire MC. Adverse reactions to neuromuscular blocking agents. Curr Allergy Asthma Rep. 2004;4:7–16.
53. Karila C, Brunet-Langot D, Labbez F, Jacqmarcq O, Ponvert C, Paupe J, et al. Anaphylaxis during anesthesia: results of a 12-year survey at a French pediatric center. Allergy. 2005;60:828–34.
54. Beaudouin E, Prestat F, Schmitt M, Kanny G, Laxenaire MC, Moneret-Vautrin DA. High risk of sensitization to latex in children with spina bifida. Eur J Pediatr Surg. 1994;4:90–3.
55. Tucke J, Posch A, Baur X, Rieger C, Rauf-Heimsoth M. Latex type I sensitization and allergy in children with atopic dermatitis evaluation of crossreactivity to some foods. Pediatr Allergy Immunol. 1999;10:160–7.
56. Berstein DI, Wanner M, Borish L, Immunotherapy Committee, American Academy of Allergy, Asthma and Immunology. Twelve-year survey of fatal reactions to allergen injections and skin testing: 1990–2001. J Allergy Clin Immunol. 2004;113:1129–36.
57. Lenchner K. Idiopathic anaphylaxis. Curr Opin Allergy Clin Immunol. 2003;3:305–11.
58. Brown A, Mckinnon D, Chu K. Emergency department anaphylaxis: a review of 142 patients in a single year. J Allergy Clin Immunol. 2001;108:861–6.
59. Pumphrey RS. Lessons for management of anaphylaxis from a study of fatal reactions. Clin Exp Allergy. 2000;30(3):1144–50.

Chapter 2
The Aetiology of Anaphylaxis

2.1 Food Allergy

2.1.1 Background

Allergy to food is a harmful reaction, involving immune mechanisms, to a foodstuff. On occasion, the harmful reaction may occur very quickly after the offending food has been swallowed, such as happens in anaphylaxis. On other occasions, a chronic reaction, like allergic eczema or allergic oesophagitis, develops. Anaphylaxis related to foods may produce dermal, gut, or respiratory symptomatology [1].

Whilst every proteinaceous component of food has an allergenic potential (and many such have been catalogued), a relatively restricted set underlies the majority of reactions. Evidence from food challenges supervised by clinicians and started off with small amounts, before increasing slowly and with adequate blinding and control in the trial, points to eggs, dairy products, groundnuts, soya bean, fish, shellfish, nuts from trees, and wheat as the most common allergens. Increasingly, sesame is implicated as an allergic trigger [2].

© Springer Nature Switzerland AG 2020
C. Cingi, N. B. Muluk, *Quick Guide to Anaphylaxis*,
https://doi.org/10.1007/978-3-030-33639-4_2

Where an anaphylactic reaction to food has caused death or near-death, it is most common to find groundnuts, nuts from trees, or shellfish being responsible, but dairy products are also implicated more and more [3].

Harmful responses to food which do not involve the immune system are not defined as allergic, a case in point being lactose intolerant patients, who have deficient lactase function. Foods may also provoke a damaging response through poisoning (such as bacterial contamination) or drug-related (such as caffeine) [2].

2.1.2   Definition of Food Allergy

"Food allergy" is the usual label employed where items in someone's dietary intake provoke an immune system response. But whilst all foods have the theoretical potential to trigger anaphylactic responses, additives such as preservatives and colouring agents rarely cause anaphylaxis. Indeed, the usual culprits in the US are as described earlier [4]. There is geographical variation in causative allergen: for instance, sesame is a frequent culprit in Israel and some other locales, but somewhat rarely so in the USA. Calculating the prevalence of food allergy is as hard as working out how common anaphylaxis (not otherwise specified) is. Self-reported food allergy occurrences of any kind, as found from surveys, give a prevalence between 3 and 35%, but these figures do not match those resulting from OFC (oral food challenges), which give prevalence of between 1 and 10.8% [5]. Age-related differences also exist in prevalence. The majority of paediatric anaphylactic cases are a result of food allergy. Both the US and the UK research data have demonstrated a doubling of groundnut allergy rates, now estimated at 1 in 100 of schoolchildren [6]. According to a report dated from 2008, authored by the US Centers for Disease Control, the 10 years from 1997 to 2007 witnessed a growth of 18% in cases of paediatric food allergy. About 3.9% of children in the USA are thought to suffer from allergy to food. Mortality associated with food allergy is especially linked to eating groundnut and tree nuts, but also has a link with either not being treated with epinephrine at all or being treated too late. In general, deaths occur most often in patients' teens or early adulthood, and where the food allergy is already known about [3, 7].

It is imperative that the patients receive written advice tailored to their situation about how to keep away from foods which are known to cause the patients an allergic reaction, not forgetting situations where the food's presence may be unmarked (and therefore harder to avoid), such as at open buffets, in meals eaten out, and in bakery and confectionery products. Signposting reliable, up-to-the-minute advice about keeping clear of the offending foods is a must [8, 9]. Strategies to keep away from certain foods can, however, make life less enjoyable for patients with a chance of anaphylaxis, due to disruptive adaptations in lifestyle and the fact that warnings on foods may be unclear and they may end up worrying about unforeseen food hazards [8, 13]. Likewise, completely steering clear of multiple foods may cause dietary insufficiencies [8]. Some of these patients, or those caring for them, may put their trust in complementary or alternative healthcare instead [14, 15].

Despite complications of anaphylaxis being unusual and death very seldom occurring, therapy as it stands has a large effect on how patients live and how good their life is [16]. The majority of allergic reactions to food begin when a child is small, and although certain allergies dwindle over time, others do not. It is thought that four fifths of patients who were allergic to dairy or egg as children can eat these safely by the age of 16 [17, 18], and groundnut allergy, typically considered a permanent situation, now appears to remit without intervention in up to a fifth of elementary school-aged sufferers [6]. On the other hand, reports suggest that peanuts may elicit a reaction afresh even when OFC was negative, and they had been excluded successfully from the diet [6, 7].

At the time of writing, no curative treatments exist. Given the upheaval food allergy diagnoses may cause to patients and relatives, getting the diagnosis right is vital. Food allergies are diagnosed along the same lines as other allergies, as described earlier. Dermal prick tests and laboratory IgE titres can give an idea about sensitivities, but in the end OFC might well be needed to ensure accuracy. To conduct an OFC, progressively larger doses of the putative offending food substance are administered. A doctor needs to be on hand, and the test should only happen where adequate resuscitation facilities for anaphylaxis are available, with practitioners skilled in dealing with anaphylaxis in attendance. The ideal way of diagnosing food allergy is still a double-blind, placebo-controlled OFC (DBPCFC), but open trials or ones with one party unaware of allocations remain common [19]. Given that a DBPCFC may give a falsely negative outcome, in such cases, the potentially problematic food should be fed once more, unmasked, but with resuscitation available [7, 19, 20].

A diagnosis of anaphylaxis linked to a food leads directly to therapy based on that food's elimination from the diet. The sufferer, their relatives, and those caring for them need to be instructed on how to pay attention to food labelling in the preparation of meals and consider how safe food eaten outside the home is, as well as the need to avoid transfer of antigens whilst making meals, such as from kitchenware used repeatedly. Simpler terminology on food labels is now mandated by US law. Thus "casein" is now labelled "milk". However, since the range of allergens so described is limited (mainly milk, eggs, wheat, soya, groundnut, tree nuts, fish, and shellfish), it does not make other allergens any easier to pick out. Alert bands and wearable tags need to be recommended to patients and those caring for them, and they should be able to spot anaphylaxis warning signs and deal with them as they occur. Writing an action plan specific to the patient is helpful for getting families ready to respond if the food is accidentally swallowed [7, 21].

2.1.3   Epidemiology

Up to 25–30% of families contain one or more food allergy sufferers, if non-specialised surveys are to be believed [22, 23]. But where the diagnosis has been made using OFC with a control, lower rates are invariably reported [2].

There is not much research available which deals with all aspects of the OFC. Rates estimated to range between 1 and

10.8% are reported from meta-analysing six studies conducted internationally but based on allergy to dairy, eggs, groundnuts, and seafood [24].

A study employing meta-analytical methods to investigate reported allergy rates to fruits and vegetables other than groundnuts ascertained only a half dozen which used OFC. These studies reported fruit and tree nut allergy prevalence as 0.1–4.3%, 0.1–1.4% for vegetables, and wheat, soya, and sesame allergies all had less than 1% prevalence [2, 25].

2.1.3.1 Sex- and Age-Related Demographics

Boys have more allergies than girls, but women outnumber men amongst adult allergy sufferers [26]. As many as 8 in 100 infants and children have a food allergy, and as many as 3.7 in 100 adults [27].

Prevalence does, nonetheless, depend on how it is calculated (patient's account, testing, doctor's evaluation), location in the world and what foods were asked about [28].

For the last 10 years, younger children have been showing an increased tendency to be allergic to foods in the UK and the USA [26, 29], according to researchers. In one case, groundnut allergy shot up from 0.4 to 0.8% between 1997 and 2002 [26]. Researchers studying Canadian and UK paediatric populations put groundnut allergy prevalence above 1% [30, 31].

A 50% increase in food allergies in those under the age of 17, from the 1997–1999 rate of 3.4% to the 2009–2011 rate of 5.1% has been reported by the US Centres for Disease Control [32].

On the basis of reported research, it has been calculated that these readily available foodstuffs have a corresponding allergy-causing rate as follows [27]:

- Cows' milk—2.5%
- Eggs—1.3%
- Groundnuts—0.8%
- Wheat—0.4%
- Soya—0.4%

2.1.4   Aetiology

Allergies mostly occur via immune responsivity to proteinaceous food components, whilst allergy to food additives of
other chemical composition remains rare [33]. In the normal
situation, oral tolerance, as it is termed, prevents the immune
system responding to food [34, 35]. This tolerance may fail, and
a maladaptive immune response occurs. But why this should be
the case is unknown, other than speculating a likely genetic or
environmental aetiology [2].

Whilst the usual scenario considered is one in which IgE is
produced following swallowing food itself, with ensuing sensitisation, other scenarios are also possible, such as in the oral allergy
syndrome (pollen-food-related syndrome), where the protein
antigens on particular uncooked fruits and vegetables have homo-
logues on pollen, and it is this pollen as inspired, not the foodstuff
in the oral cavity, that sets off the immune sensitivity. Exposure
can also possibly provoke sensitivity dermally [2, 36].

2.1.4.1   IgE Antibody-Mediated Responses

Immunoglobulin E mediates acute reactions. In addition, the type of
food reaction most often noted occurs through IgE. Atopic patients'
immune systems generate IgE specific to one or several protein
regions (known as epitopes) in a food. Basophils in the blood and
histiocytes have binding receptors for IgE with high affinity. They
are found dermally, in the gut and in the respiratory organs [2].

If the allergen is encountered at a later date, IgE will bind and
aggregate with other IgE molecules coating the cell, leading to
the receptor and the intracellular cascade being switched on,
resulting in histamine (or another signalling molecule) being
discharged and the production of pro-allergenic inflammatory
substances, such as chemotactic modulators and cytokines. The
ensuing vasodilatory, smooth muscle contractile and mucosecre-
tory response account for the observable symptoms of an acute
allergic response following food being swallowed [2].

2.1.4.2 Cell-Mediated Responses

Alongside humoral responses, cellular immune responses also occur, this mechanism being of special importance in chronic or postponed reactions. FPIES (food protein–induced enterocolitis syndrome), a reaction within the gut, seemingly depends on TNFα (the tumour necrosis factor cytokine) being synthesised by T-cells [37]. Allergic eczema sufferers sensitive to milk produce T-cells that can be shown in the laboratory to synthesise cutaneous lymphocytic antigen, which causes the response at home in dermal regions [38]. Gluten protein sensitivity by the immune system produces coeliac disease [2].

2.1.5 Symptoms of Food Allergy

Whilst the immune system ensures health through combating infection and other disease-producing processes, if food or a substance within it is incorrectly classified by the immune system as a threat, an allergy results from what would ordinarily be a beneficial response. Although the case for a genetic basis for allergy is evident, currently, it is not feasible to anticipate whether offspring or siblings of affected probands will develop a comparable condition. Research findings indicate that subsequent offspring of the parents of a child with groundnut allergy may also develop the condition. Allergic responses run the full gamut of seriousness. An initially mild response is a poor predictor of the severity of subsequent responses, thus a subsequent reaction may be characterised by a more severe symptomatology [39].

At the most extreme end of the spectrum of severity lies anaphylaxis, a potentially lethal systemic allergic response causing respiratory compromise, acute hypotension, and tachycardia. Onset is possible within minutes of antigenic exposure, and since death can occur, timely administration of epinephrine is essential.

All foods have the potential to provoke an adverse response, but in fact, 90% of anaphylactic reactions are attributable to just eight food types [39]:

- Eggs
- Milk
- Peanuts
- Tree nuts
- Fish
- Shellfish
- Wheat
- Soy

In addition, there are some seeds (such as sesame and mustard—the principal ingredient in table mustard) which are frequently implicated in food allergies and constitute a principal cause in some territories [39].

Allergic symptomatology can be cutaneous, gut-related, and affect the cardiovascular and respiratory organ systems. Symptoms can be evident as at least one of [39]:

- Emesis plus or minus griping.
- Urticaria.
- Dyspnoea.
- Cardiovascular shock.
- Laryngeal constriction and voice alteration; dysphagia.
- Glossoedema with airway compromise.
- Indistinct pulse.
- Cyanosis.
- Syncope and dizziness.
- Anaphylaxis, which can be lethal, causing respiratory compromise and cardiovascular shock. Symptoms may occur within distinct organ systems concurrently, such as cutaneous rash with gastric pain.
- Itching of the mouth and pharynx.
- Blood vessel inflammation (swelling of larynx).
- Extra sounds when breathing.
- Altered voice.

- Loud breathing.
- Feeling nauseous.
- Loose stools.
- Going red in the head and neck region.
- Red eyes, itching of the eyes, swelling of the conjunctivae, swelling around the eye.
- Blocked nose, itching nose, runny nose, and sneezing.
- Abdominodynia.
- Angor mortis.
- Cardiovascular compromise [2].

A complete history needs to encompass [2]:

- All suspected food triggers
- Format of food (uncooked, cooked, extra elements)
- How much food seems to need to be ingested before a reaction occurs
- How reliably exposure to the food culprit provokes reaction
- Individual or family atopic tendencies
- Potentiating factors for allergy, such as exercise [40], NSAIDs (non-steroidal anti-inflammatory drugs), alcoholic consumption

As well, a detailed, comprehensive account should be noted for every allergic response, not forgetting:

- The way the exposure occurred (swallowing, dermal, respiratory) and amount
- Temporal relationship between exposure and beginning of reaction
- Catalogue of symptomatology with indication of severity
- How long the reaction persisted
- Therapeutic responses and effectiveness or otherwise
- Latest allergic response

The physical aims to inform a judgement as to:

- How well-nourished and how developed physically the patient is and what stigmata of allergic disease are present
- Exclusion of conditions with extensive mimicry for allergic problems

The majority of symptoms linked to allergic responses to food happen within a 2 h time frame, but many have a much shorter time frame. A time frame lasting more than 4–6 h, whilst possible, is seldom encountered, but if this does happen, the patient may be a child with allergic dermatitis secondary to food or the seldom seen red meat allergy following being bitten by lone star ticks [39].

FPIES can cause a different type of allergic reaction with a delayed onset. It is a reaction within the gut beginning 1 or 2 h post ingestion of milk, soya, a few types of grain, and certain solid foods. Peak occurrence is in young children under 1 year of age for whom these foods are new or who are in the process of weaning. It may provoke multiple vomiting episodes and may cause the patient to become dehydrated. On occasion, babies may have blood mixed in with prolific loose stools. Due to its resemblance to a viral or bacterial infection, it may take some time for FPIES to be diagnosed; however, the sequelae are serious enough to warrant emergency treatment and intravenous resuscitation [39].

Symptoms linked to certain foods need not indicate the presence of an allergy nor necessitate absolute elimination from the diet; an example would be patients who experience oral pruritus following consumption of raw or uncooked fruits or vegetables, since such a picture may represent oral allergy syndrome, caused not by the food but by pollen. An epitopic similarity between pollen and food proteins initiates an allergic response, except where cooking abolishes the similarity, rendering the food harmless [39].

2.1.6   Food Allergy Triggers

If food allergy has been diagnosed, the treatment of choice is elimination of the food from the diet. The following foods have a strong association with paediatric food allergy cases:

- Milk
- Eggs
- Groundnuts

Whilst a child may lose the milk or egg allergic response, groundnut and tree nuts usually continue to provoke symptoms.

Amongst adults, the usual culprits are [39]:

- Pollen from fruits and vegetables in cases of oral allergy syndrome
- Groundnuts and tree nuts
- Fish and shellfish

Some degree of allergic cross-reactivity is observable amongst related foods, thus sensitivity to one tree nut may predispose to allergy towards others, or prawn allergy may co-occur with crab and lobster sensitivity. Groundnuts are in fact legumes rather than true nuts, so, whilst groundnut allergy being cross-reactive with walnuts, almonds, and cashews is well known, the seldom encountered cross-reactivity with other legumes (but not soya) makes botanical sense. This is an argument for specialist treatment by a qualified expert on allergology, since cross-reactivity needs to be explained and taught to the patient. It is a non-trivial matter to determine cross reactivity. Even where a number of potential problem foods within a grouping have been tested for, there may be a lack of specificity, since the test lacks discriminatory power to distinguish between in-group items. Evidence of having eaten an item without problems in the past can signify that a cross-reactivity in theory in practice does not apply, and the food can continue being eaten. On the other hand, if the test is negative, possible allergic problems related to that item can be discounted. If testing shows reactivity for previously unencountered foodstuffs which are within a grouping, some of whose members have been eaten before and caused a problem, the ideal way to manage the risk is OFC [39].

2.1.7 Diagnosing Food Allergies

It is usual for allergenic items to produce symptoms on all occasions when encountered. There is, however, inter- and intra-individual variation in symptomatology. Allergic symptoms may be cutaneous, affecting breathing, the gut or the heart, and circulation. Foreseeing the severity of a particular reaction is not achievable; hence, all cases of food allergy require meticulous attention to advising the sufferer about the potential for anaphylaxis, which carries the risk of mortality and necessitates epinephrine (adrenaline) administration.

The peak occurrence of food allergy is when the patient remains a young child, but onset occurs throughout the lifespan. Where food allergy appears possible, consultation with an allergology clinician, involving history-taking focused on both the patient and family members, followed by testing if appropriate, precedes confirmation or exclusion of the food allergy diagnosis.

An allergy history focuses on both symptomatology and other health issues. Patients need to be ready to respond to enquiry concerning:

- Identity of food trigger and quantity
- Latent period before symptoms emerged
- Enumeration of symptoms and duration of each

Following the documentation of symptoms, cutaneous testing with or without immunoglobulin E serology may be needed [39]:

- Cutaneous testing lasts approximately 20 min and involves the cutaneous application of antigen suspended in solution. Liquid gains entry under the skin following the introduction of a small calibre probing device into the skin, using aseptic technique. It is generally of mild painfulness, and the development of a raised area on the overlying skin (appearances mimic those of mosquito bites) indicates a positive result. A negative control performs the same procedure without using the antigen in solution, leading to no wheal formation. Sites are thus visibly different.

- Serology lacks the specificity of dermal testing, and titres are recorded for IgE reactive to epitopes on the suspected item. Serology takes up to 1 week and is quantitative.

Allergologists need to take account of testing before diagnosing food allergy, but positive testing need not always lead to diagnosis of food allergy, whereas negative testing does exclude the possibility. On occasion, OFC, the gold standard in diagnosis, will be felt necessary, in the course of which minute quantities of the potential allergenic food are administered, increasing the amount stepwise, to the patient over a certain period. A clinician must be in attendance, and the observation continues after cessation of testing for up to several hours. OFC is of particular relevance where history lacks clarity or if dermal testing and serology are ambiguous. OFC may also confirm where a sufferer no longer exhibits symptoms and tolerance has developed.

Given the risk-laden nature of the procedure, OFC should occur only where a clinic has the services of clinicians specialised in allergology and is equipped with facilities for urgent resuscitation [39].

The following pathology investigations may be of benefit [2]:

- IgE serology for allergen-particular antibodies: if positive, the patient has been sensitised to an antigen, but this does not invariably translate into a clinically observable allergic response. Certain sensitivities lack an appropriate assay.
- Histamine-release assay (basophils). For the most part, restricted to the research area.

Dermal tests of interest are:

- Prick test: the test ordered with the highest frequency in food allergy, although can predict absence of allergy (>90% accurate) more reliably than presence (<50%)
- Intradermal test: hazardous due to possibility of initiating systemic involvement and therefore rarely used
- Patch test: initial results encouraging, however not yet suitable for everyday clinical use

Diagnosis can also be supported by recording or adjusting the diet:

- Record of food eaten (diary)
- Dietary avoidance (both as treatment and to aid diagnosis)
- Challenge of offending item, open or single- or double-blinded, with placebo

2.1.8   Characteristics of Food Allergens

A typical dietary allergen is a glycoprotein with a molecular mass between 10,000 and 70,000 daltons, soluble in water and capable of resisting thermal degradation and proteolytic attack. Thus it can be readily absorbed through a mucosa. Many dietary allergens have been isolated and their molecular characteristics extensively delineated, e.g. Ara h1-3 (groundnut origin), Gal d1-3 (chicken egg albumen-derived), Gly m1 (soyabean husks), Gad c1 (fish), and Pen a1 (prawns).

Foods which are similar often produce similar allergens that in turn lead to measurable quantities of particular IgE on serology or dermal testing. However, clinically speaking, allergic cross-reactivity across similar foods is less common [41]. Allergic reactivity to meat-derived proteins which occurs after a delay may be attributable to a carbohydrate moiety being the epitope [2, 42].

2.1.9   Risk Factors

Anaphylaxis leading to death is an especial risk in patients who:

1. Are asthmatic, more so if the disease is not under adequate control.
2. Have had an anaphylactic reaction as a result of that item in the past.
3. Had early warning signs missed.
4. Were not immediately administered epinephrine, or where there was no epinephrine to hand [3, 43].

5. Are teenage or in early adulthood. This last group is in fact especially at risk and their deaths are higher than expected in registries of deaths secondary to food allergy.

2.1.10 Management and Treatment

The principal strategy for dealing with a food allergy involves eliminating the problem food from the diet. Food labelling requires special attention by the patient, note being taken of alternative ways of listing a problem food. In the USA, it is a requirement of The Food Allergy Labeling and Consumer Protection Act of 2004 (FALCPA) for producers of food contained in packaging that, if the ingredients include at least one of the eight principal allergenic foods, even if only as a minor ingredient, additive or flavouring, the label must reflect the presence in an evident way that is not open to misunderstanding. These eight foods are dairy, egg, wheat, soya, groundnut, tree nut, fish, and crustaceans [39].

Additionally, warnings about possible contamination with allergenic substances may be affixed to products, worded as "may/ might contain", "produced in a factory making", etc., but such advice notices are not stipulated legally, nor do standards for them exist. It should be noted that the FALCPA regulations do not cover items, the regulation of which lies under a different agency, such as the Department of Agriculture (meat, poultry, and some egg-containing items) or alcoholic beverages (Alcohol and Tobacco Tax and Trade Bureau). Cosmetic items, shampoo, and health and beauty products may all contain ingredients derived from tree nuts or wheat, but labelling legislation does not apply to them [39].

Eliminating contact with allergens is easy in theory, but difficult in practice. Despite the benefits of clear labelling, the ubiquity of some ingredients makes avoidance an uphill task. The assistance of specialists in diet or nutrition, who can balance avoidance of allergen with maintaining an adequate diet, may prove of benefit. Support groups, both face-to-face and virtual, and specialised recipe books, targeted towards allergy sufferers, are potential sources of knowledge. A frequently asked question concerns whether an allergy may abate, but the answer is currently debatable. However, one set of allergies (milk, eggs, wheat, soya) has a greater tendency to abate than the other (groundnut, tree nuts, fish, and shellfish).

Additional precautions are needed when eating out, as food service (and occasionally food preparation) personnel may lack familiarity with the ingredients used over the whole choice offered. In extreme cases, the mere act of entering a food service or preparation area may provoke allergic symptoms. An expedient, available online from many sites, is a "chef card", containing pertinent details of a sufferer's allergies. Sufferers should be encouraged to advise food service staff about allergies and, where practicable, inform the chef directly, emphasising the necessity for a food preparation area and equipment free from allergenic contamination and identifying which menu items entail the least risk [39].

Allergen-specific oral immunotherapy aimed at blocking anaphylaxis due to food at present remains at the development phase, but clinical trials involving the enrolment of sufferers from milk, egg, and groundnut allergies have been initiated in centres of excellence for the treatment and investigation of allergy (using OFC and immunotherapy) and anaphylaxis [44–52]. A proportion of such investigational trials conform to a blinded RCT design. Side effect incidence thus far remains high with certain immunotherapy regimens, notably whilst the dosage is being increased on Day 1 and at later dose increment stages [53].

A number of researchers report that clinically observable removal of food-related allergic sensitivity correlates with ongoing serological and cellular adjustments [50, 52] reflected in lower positivity to dermal prick tests, basophilic activation reduction, lessened IgE titres with higher recorded titres for IgG_4, CSIF, interferon gamma, and TNF-α [52]. Research under way addresses the question of the extent to which clinically observable tolerance translates into a genuine immunological tolerance, whereby sufferers can encounter the allergen after a long absence from the diet without a resurgence in symptoms [45–47].

Research based on specific immunotherapy to dietary and other allergens is likely to focus in the future on sublingual allergenic desensitisation, genetically modified proteins using recombinant DNA (or mixtures composed thereof), CpG motif oligodeoxynucleotides complexed with allergens, allergoids (peptides or other polymers), and various remaining innovatory approaches [45].

Ways to modulate the immune system as a whole are similarly under research. A combination of Chinese medicinal plants known as Food Allergy Herbal Formula-2, of known chemical composition, can block anaphylaxis secondary to food and induces durable immunotolerance in mice and is in the clinical trial phase [54]. There is a possibility that anti-IgE immunoglobulins injected subcutaneously may reduce the risk of food- or other allergen-induced anaphylactic reactions for a sizeable number (but not all) of sufferers [15, 55].

Nonetheless, at the time of writing, disease-modifying agents for food allergy remain in the future, and the mainstay of treatment is absolute avoidance of ingestion of known allergens. Such a regime, if adequately implemented and nutritionally complete, comprises [2]:

- Training sufferers and their relatives to read labels on foodstuffs and reliably note if a term used refers to the allergen(s) at issue
- Ensuring contamination with allergen during cooking does not occur, from kitchen equipment used for different items
- Avoidance of all sources of allergens, both overt and covert (e.g. in medicines or makeup), but not avoidance of non-allergenic foodstuffs
- Monitoring of other ways in which antigen may be encountered (e.g. breathing in substance or it touching patient's skin)
- Planning ahead to keep clear of potential cross-reactive sources, e.g. groundnuts and lupines, or milk from different animals [41]

- Not getting into the risk of encountering the antigen by accident or without realising it, such as eating from buffets or attending picnics.

Despite such measures, antigen may still be eaten without the patient realising or by ill-luck. Thus there also needs to be a plan in place for an appropriate response in such a case:

- Written documentation of what to do in brief but accurate way, readily accessible in places where sufferer is likely to be (creche, school, workplace, hall of residence) to responsible individuals
- Wearing of medalert bands, tags, etc. with allergy stated
- Ensuring availability of emergency contact number
- Training patient in advance of an emergency, such as common ways in which unintended antigenic exposure may occur

2.1.10.1   Investigational Therapeutic Interventions for Food Allergy

The outlook for emerging treatments for anaphylaxis due to food remains positive. Until now, the approaches investigated include subcutaneous immunotherapy (SCIT), oral immunotherapy (OIT), sublingual immunotherapy (SLIT), and epicutaneous immunotherapy (EPIT). Other approaches that look set to be useful include traditional Chinese medicine (TCM) and monoclonal antibody administration [7].

2.1.10.2   Patient Education

Preparation

Sufferers should have self-administerable injectable epinephrine on them at all times, and it must have been stored appropriately and be within date. The method of administration and the circumstances in which use is required need to be taught carefully to the sufferer. An H1 antihistamine (as a syrup or chewable) needs to be carried, and it must have been appropriately stored and be within date. If anaphylaxis does occur, medical assistance should be sought without delay. Those looking after child sufferers need training in spotting warning signs of anaphylaxis and administering the treatment [2].

Avoidance of Allergens

Food allergy sufferers need instruction in recognition of the antigenic foodstuffs at issue, so as to allow avoidance in the diet [2], and this should include how to interpret food labelling and asking about what food contains when eating catered meals. An attitude of avoidance of an item where doubt exists should be inculcated and an awareness of hidden dangers in medicines and beauty products should be developed [2].

2.1.11 Anaphylaxis

Food allergy reactions cover the full spectrum from minor to potentially lethal, and where on the spectrum a reaction will be situated is speculative at best. A history of minor reactions does not preclude the sudden emergence of anaphylaxis, which may lead to respiratory compromise and acute hypotension. This situation explains the reluctance of allergy specialists to grade patients as "mildly" or "severely" allergic to food. The prognosis is simply too unclear. Within the community, food is the principal trigger for anaphylaxis within the US [39].

Treatment of anaphylaxis always begins with epinephrine. Anaphylaxis itself can be defined as shock induced by an immune chemical cascade. The time between exposure and first symptoms may be a few minutes or less and may progress with extreme rapidity and threaten life. Upon first diagnosis of food allergy, epinephrine should be prescribed for auto-injection. A documented treatment plan listing current drug history and indications should be supplied. Patients should check expiry dates for epinephrine and note them on their calendar plus consider using an automatic renewal service as offered by many pharmacies. Food allergy mandates the sufferer to keep the epinephrine readily available continually together with a second dose in case of recurrence of a severe reaction, as occurs in 20% of cases. Since individuals who are susceptible to second recurrence are not yet an identifiable group, the recommendation applies to food allergy sufferers across the board [39].

Dyspnoea, coughing repeatedly, barely perceptible pulse, urticaria, pharyngeal constriction, difficulty in drawing breath, or dysphagia should lead to epinephrine injection without delay, as should a pattern of symptoms arising from different organ systems, e.g. urticaria, cutaneous oedema, or rash in association with emesis, abdominodynia, and diarrhoea. A single dose may be insufficient. Either the patient or a bystander needs to summon an ambulance, alerting ambulance control of the use of epinephrine and advising that further epinephrine should be available. Attendance at accident and emergency is necessary, but local policies vary as to extent of post-administration supervision. In cases where the diagnosis may not be fully clear, the risks of superfluous administration are somewhat lower than those of non-administration [39].

Frequently encountered adverse effects of epinephrine include anxiety, agitation, lightheadedness, and tremulousness, whilst dysrhythmia, tachycardia, myocardial infarction, acute hypertension, and right-sided heart failure are seldom encountered. Comorbid conditions, e.g. diabetes mellitus or cardiac disease, may predispose to greater adverse event susceptibility secondary to epinephrine. However, the overall risk profile is favourable and has the highest efficacy amongst agents used to treat severe allergic complications. Whilst other agents are in use, none can adequately stand in for epinephrine, which alone can switch off the potentially lethal allergic response [39].

The emergency armamentarium in anaphylaxis comprises [2]:

- Epinephrine via injection, which is the best medication for treatment initially of food-related anaphylaxis. Patients need an auto-injector on their person continually and know how to use it correctly.
- Histamine blockers treat less severe symptoms.

- Bronchodilators find usage but are not sufficient in anaphylaxis, for which epinephrine is essential.
- H2 blockade may be useful in conjunction with other therapy, as may be glucocorticoids.
- Intravenous infusion to counter hypotension.
- Glucagon for anaphylaxis that is not responding to treatment.

Where anaphylactic symptoms are severe, fluid resuscitation and assisted ventilatory support are sometimes required.

Immunotherapy administered via ingestion or sublingually is an upcoming treatment of high potential value [56, 57].

2.1.12   Food Allergy Action Plan

Food allergy can adversely affect how good the sufferer's life is and limit lifestyle. Relatives describe difficulties meeting as families, going on school excursions, attending celebrations, sleeping away from home, and playing with other children [16]. A significant number of parents reduce their concerns by curtailing the child's socialising as a whole, stopping the child from going to celebrations or school excursions [58, 59]. Child sufferers also state that they are afraid about being exposed to allergens. Going to shops, eating in restaurants, and birthday celebrations may scare children for whom these activities may seem deadly [16, 60]. The inability to offer a prognosis regarding future severity of reactions leads sufferers and their caregivers to be apprehensive that a future reaction may result in death. Anaphylaxis is most often secondary to food allergy outside hospital, and food allergy numbers keep going up [61]. Whilst eliminating the antigen from the diet can stop anaphylaxis occurring, in fact other unintended contact may still happen [7].

2.1.13   Prognosis

As a rule, the majority of infants and young children develop out of an allergic state towards particular foods or become less susceptible to symptoms. Dairy, egg, soya, and wheat allergies may be left behind, but groundnut, tree nut, fish, and shellfish allergies usually remain with the patient [62].

Eighty-five percent of child milk or egg allergy sufferers develop out of the allergic state by age 3–5, according to general incidence studies [62]. Nonetheless, in a specialist setting, research indicates lower rates of outgrowth of dairy, egg, and soya allergies, such that a mere 50% of sufferers have lost symptoms of allergy by age 8–12 [63–65]. Allergies continue to be outgrown into adolescence.

At the age at which school begins, around 20% of sufferers no longer have a groundnut allergy [2].

The paediatric non-IgE-modulated allergic responses to food, e.g. procto- and entero-colitis, usually abate within the first few years of life [66]. Allergic eosinophilic oesophagitis seems to continue through life [67].

Anaphylaxis of a severe kind, with associated lethality, may be triggered by swallowing food [43]. Very marked oedema of the larynx, spasm of the bronchi that cannot be reversed, and low blood pressure not responsive to treatment or several factors together account for these deaths. The food triggers linked most frequently to severe anaphylaxis are groundnuts, tree nuts, fish, and shellfish, but many other triggers are documented. Documentation of dairy allergy occasioning fatal anaphylaxis has increased [3].

2.2   Drug Allergy

2.2.1   Definition of Drug Allergy

No drug exists that is free from side effects (often referred to as "adverse drug reactions"), but these adverse reactions are of several different types, not just allergic-type. Sometimes the reaction is idiosyncratic, has features which merely mimic an allergic response, or arises from a patient not being able to tolerate the drug. According to The British Society for Allergy and Clinical Immunology (BSACI), a drug allergy is an adverse drug reaction with an established immunological mechanism. Clinically this mechanism may not be evident, and deciding if a particular reaction constitutes an allergy may necessitate investigating more deeply [68].

A 2003 definition of "drug allergy" by the World Allergy Association (WAO) states that hypersensitivity must be present, and this should depend on immune involvement. Both IgE-modulated and non-IgE (principally involving T-cells) subtypes exist [69, 70].

The reason for admitting a patient to hospital in 3–6% of cases is an adverse drug event, and whilst in hospital, 10–15% of patients overall also experience the same, hence adverse drug reactions cause increased morbidity, longer hospital stays, and deaths. The World Health Organisation (WHO) offers the following explanation of ADR: "a response to a medicine which is noxious and unintended, and which occurs at doses normally used in man" [71].

The majority (80%) of ADRs are type A, where they can be anticipated and are linked to dosage. An example is bleeding into the gut following NSAIDs (non-steroidal anti-inflammatories) and other unwanted effects predictable from pharmacological mechanisms. The remaining 15–20% are type B, which cannot be anticipated and are not tied to dosage. Included within type B are both allergies (immune-dependent hypersensitivity) and other idiosyncratic types (non-immune in nature) [72].

The SCAR category (Severe Cutaneous Adverse Reaction) encompasses Stevens–Johnson syndrome (SJS), toxic epidermal necrolysis (TEN) [73–77], drug-induced hypersensitivity syndrome (DiHS), and drug rash with eosinophilia and systemic symptoms (DRESS) [78]. A new arrival to the SCAR category is acute generalised exanthematous pustulosis (AGEP) [79, 80]. Drugs also frequently precipitate an anaphylactic reaction [69, 83]. Anaphylaxis is severe and potentially lethal and affects the whole body [81, 82].

Drug allergies occur where a patient who has previously been sensitised to a drug formulation (active agent or excipient) subsequently has a reaction of his/her immune system to that drug.

Categorising types of allergy is hampered by an incomplete picture of the true pathophysiology. The Gell–Coombs scheme was previously of benefit, but we now know many common types do not fit the scheme. Since a replacement is lacking, the version in use, incorporating modifications, is still of some value in certain cases. The abundant research literature on allergy to penicillin has yielded most of the current insights into IgE's role in drug allergy as a whole, but the picture from other studies is slowly appearing although so far not in great depth. Non-IgE-mediated allergies are better understood, as are adverse reactions in general such as aspirin-exacerbated respiratory disease (AERD) [84].

2.2.2   Classification of Drug Allergy

Allergic responses to drugs can be categorised by means of the Gell–Coombs scheme of immune types in man: type I (IgE dependent), type II (toxic to living cells), type III (complexes formed), and type IV (non-humoral, cell-based). A subtype of type IV is reactions that occur after a delay and are cellular-based.

A classification put forward recently for type IV reactions proposes the cell populations involved as a way to separate types, thus IVa to IVd involve, respectively, monocytes, eosinophils, T-cells (CD4 or CD8 lineages), and neutrophils [85]. The archetypal type IV reaction is eczematous, completely confined to the cutaneous system and occasioned by an allergic sensitisation primed initially and then provoked by exposure to a drug. Seemingly, Gell–Coombs type IV mechanisms underlie the skin rashes that appear after a delay, for example the maculopapular exanthemata secondary to antimicrobials (especially amoxicillin and the sulphonamides) and toxic pustuloderma. A further way to divide drug allergy occurrences is by principal site affected (whole body, skin, liver), a pragmatic option that gets around the problems of isolating a putative immunological characterisation. There is a range of allergic reactions and clinical entities that can occur with drugs [84]. A more detailed discussion follows.

Researchers have newly put forward a further classification scheme to address the variety of drug-related hypersensitivity types. It is termed p-i ("pharmacological interaction with immune receptor"). A drug is visualised as entering into a non-covalent interaction with receptors located on T-cells, enabling immunoreactivity through subsequent activation of an MHC receptor. This conceptual schema does away with the need for a pre-existing sensitisation event, as the involvement of T-cells (memory and effector) is induced directly, similarly to how superantigens work [86, 87]. Whilst consideration of the structure of a drug may, in some cases, allow prediction of which type of hypersensitivity is likely to result, such as with penicillin or the peptides, this is not universally so. Characteristics of the drug antigen linked to risk are dosage, way given, length of treatment, recurrent exposures, and comorbidities. Patient risk factors involve sex, age, allergic diathesis, possession of certain alleles, and multiple drug allergy syndrome (a tendency to have a reaction to many drugs of various kinds that is constitutional) [84].

2.2.3   Epidemiology

How common drug allergy is remains unclear. For the most part, pharmacoepidemiological studies have focused on ADRs in general rather than specifically allergic reactions to drugs [88] and are restricted to specified subpopulations, such as in- or out-patients visiting Accident and Emergency, family practice settings or specialist clinics for allergology, adults or children, patients with skin reactions in general or SCAR (severe cutaneous adverse reactions) [89], or anaphylaxis of whatever cause as a single diagnosis.

To diagnose an adverse reaction and implicate a particular drug, most of this research employs the ADR definitions provided by the WHO. How SCAR was defined and subtyped in the 1980s through to early 1990s and differs from later classifications. Moreover, the bulk of research confined to drug allergy itself was dependent upon an account substantiating a time relationship between the beginning of drug use and the beginning of symptoms, together with a clinical presentation pointing towards a drug reaction. Few studies or data collections [90] came from standardised clinical patient surveys [91] or corroborated the diagnosis by means of in vivo or in vitro testing [92–94].

In the 5 years up to 2000, there were 62,000 occasions annually in England on which a patient suffering from a drug allergy or other ADR was hospitalised, according to the Hospital Episode Statistics. It also appears that the incidence is going up: in 2005 serious ADRs were at 2.6 times the level of 1998 [95]. Approaching 15% of those in hospital stay longer than anticipated following an ADR. Approximately 0.5 million patients in UK state hospitals carry a drug allergy diagnosis, the majority of which are penicillin-allergic. Around 1 in 10 people in general assert that they are allergic to penicillin [96], frequently due to recalling a dermal eruption in the course of paediatric treatment with the antibiotic, but in fact, those genuinely penicillin allergic do not even represent 10% of such people [96]. As a result, 9% of the population may be considered non-allergic to penicillin [97, 98].

Research indicates that possessing a diagnosis of penicillin allergy renders a patient more liable to treatment with broad spectrum antibiotics (quinolones, vancomycin, third-generation cephalosporins) [99], which then carries the risk of more frequent iatrogenic complications, e.g. antibiotic treatment resistance and *Clostridium difficile* infection, with concomitantly prolonged hospitalisation [100].

Critical care patients found to host vancomycin-resistant enterococci (VRE) had a fivefold increased incidence of treatment with vancomycin and third-generation cephalosporin within the preceding month compared with controls [101]. Penicillin allergy lacking substantive proof thus can mean broad-spectrum antibiotics other than penicillins get misused, resulting in bacterial resistant strains emerging and less effective therapeutic choices being made [68].

NSAIDs (non-steroidal anti-inflammatory drugs), including ibuprofen, diclofenac, naproxen, and aspirin, frequently provoke hypersensitivity reactions [98, 102]. The rate amongst asthmatic patients is between 1 in 20 and 1 in 10, whilst patients with chronic hives have a 1 in 3 chance of a severe reaction (angio-edema or anaphylaxis) to NSAID use [103, 104]. Anaphylaxis has a general prevalence of 0.1%, whilst its prevalence under general anaesthesia is once per 10–20,000 anaesthetic administrations [105, 106]. It may prove necessary to prevent such patients from receiving a general anaesthetic in future, supposing safe drug selections cannot be identified [68, 107].

2.2.4 Drug Allergy and Anaphylaxis

Salvo et al. undertook a review of computerised records dating from 1988 to 2006 and pertaining to ADRs following giving drugs by mouth. These records were generated from spontaneous reporting to the Italian Interregional Group of Pharmacovigilance (GIF) by seven different parts of Italy [108]. The definition of drug allergy employed was anaphylactic shock or anaphylactoid symptoms, skin or whole body (at least two separate organs or systems) reactions and a period between administration and beginning of symptoms compatible with an allergic reaction. The length of this period, however, was not specified. ADR reports were screened by toxicologists, clinical pharmacologists, and pharmacists as needed and totalled 27,175. About 3143 met the criteria for drug allergy, some 11.6% of total ADRs. The RORs (reported odds ratios) that reached statistical significance were for antibiotics (2.92, 95% CI 2.71, 3.15) and NSAIDs (1.65, 95% CI 1.51, 1.81) as the cause of the allergy. For antibiotics, cinoxacin and moxifloxacin had the highest RORs (6.88, 95% CI 4.19, 11.29 and 4.20, 95% CI 3.19, 5.55, respectively). For NSAIDs, compounds derived from propionate, especially ibuprofen, held the highest RORs. These were 2.75 (95% CI 2.30, 3.28) for propionate derivatives and 4.2 (95% CI 3.13, 5.63) for ibuprofen [69].

The absence of agreement on how to define anaphylaxis, the different types of populations researched plus the divergent techniques of collecting the data have all contributed to the difficulty in quantifying the prevalence or incidence of anaphylaxis. In the West, perhaps some 8–50 cases of anaphylaxis occur in every 100,000 person-years, and over a lifetime, individuals have a 0.05–2% chance of an anaphylactic episode [109]. But this is at best an estimate, and true figures for this, as well as for deaths arising from drug-related anaphylaxis, remain out of reach.

Drugs feature prominently amongst the causes of anaphylaxis occurring due to IgE-linked mechanisms, especially penicillin and anaesthetic agents, uncovered by such research. For anaphylaxis not due to allergy, NSAIDs and radio-contrast agents were often the culprit. The age range 55–84 had the highest risk of anaphylaxis due to drugs (3.8 per 100,000 people). Males under 15 were affected more than females in Australia [110]. In three countries, of the deaths due to anaphylaxis most were linked to drug allergy—the United Kingdom [111], New Zealand [112], and Australia [113].

During the 1960s and 1970s, penicillin was held to be the most frequent trigger for drug-related anaphylaxis in the USA [114, 115], but the following decades have not produced corroborative figures from pharmacoepidemiology to back this up [116]. Drugs administered perioperatively also achieve prominence according to a number of studies from all across the globe. The combined incidence of both immune and other mechanism acute hypersensitivity to anaesthesia has been reported as follows: 1 in 5000–13,000 in Australia [117], 1 in 4600 in France [118], 1 in 5000 in Thailand [119], 1 in 1250–5000 in New Zealand, and 1 in 3500 in England [120]. For hypersensitivity occurring through immune mechanisms, most frequently resulting from use of either neuromuscular blockade or antibiotic administration [69, 122], the rates were: 1 in 10,000–20,000 in Australia [117], 1 in 13,000 in France [118], 1 in 10,263 in Spain, 1 in 5500 in Thailand [119], and 1 in 1700–20,000 in Norway [121].

2.2.5 Risk Factors for Drug Allergy

2.2.5.1 Drug-Related Factors

Certain features of a drug influence how immunogenic it is, such as whether it can perform as a hapten or prohapten, or itself form covalent bonds with receptors on immune cells (the so-called Pi concept) [123] so, as result, some drug classes are more antigenic than others [85]. How the drug is given also has an apparent effect: given without a break, the same drug appears less prone to sensitising the patient than when given at intervals and repeatedly, and oral administration creates fewer problems in this respect than parenteral routes. But confirmation of these findings awaits firm scientific validation [69].

2.2.5.2 Factors Related to the Host

Female humans are seemingly more at risk of drug allergy than males, but the effect may be linked to the general female predilection of ADRs. Females outnumbered males by 2 to 1 in being seen at initial presentation for a drug allergy, according to the Alergológica 2005 study [124]. In addition, females usually outnumbered males in reporting allergies to drugs by their own reckoning [125]. Different research reveals that drug allergies affect more women than men [126, 127]. Hospital registry data indicate that woman inpatients had a greater likelihood of developing drug allergies than their male counterparts at the level of statistical significance, but how this manifested clinically and how often it resulted in death revealed no differences between groups [128]. Currently, it remains an unresolved issue whether drug allergies are genuinely fewer in children [129, 130]. Despite an absence for children of repeated exposures to drugs, an essential element in sensitisation, the fact that some particular drugs are prescribed very widely in this group may suggest the possibility of sensitisation occurring in a subgroup, such as chronic disease sufferers, who may get repeated batches of antibiotics.

ADRs go up as patients' age, as do admissions to hospital resulting from ADRs; however, what relationship exists between age and drug allergy has been less extensively researched [130]. How drug allergy presents and what happens as a result are similar in both elderly and younger inpatients, but the graver type of response (anaphylaxis, SJS, TEN, DiHS) is less frequently seen amongst the elderly [69, 131].

Comorbid disorders may facilitate allergic drug hypersensitivity responses through metabolic alterations and by widening the scope for immune-mediated responses. In the case of SLE, however, a seeming rise in drug allergy occurrences has not been borne out by the data in a reliable fashion [132]. Patients in receipt of antiretroviral therapy for HIV commonly have drug allergies to particular agents, e.g. cotrimoxazole, abacavir, and nevirapine, and it is thought probable that immune reconstitution and the genetic makeup of the patient lay the grounds for such allergic hypersensitivity [133]. In an analogous fashion, DiHS may be linked to occasions when herpesviridae (Epstein–Barr virus, human herpes virus 6 and 7, and cytomegalovirus) become reactivated [134]. An allergic diathesis, though, seemingly does not increase a patient's risk of developing drug allergy in a highly significant way [127]. Ethnopharmacological and pharmacogenetic factors of rising importance in predisposing patients to allergic responses to some particular classes of drugs will be outlined in the next section [69].

2.2.6 Genetics of Drug Allergy

Contemporary medical geneticists are occupied with clarifying the relationships between HLA genotype and severity of drug allergy. HLA receptors show antigenic stimuli to the TCR (T-cell receptor) on the T-cell outer membrane, which provokes an immune response. Class I of the HLA receptor family (HLA A, HLA B, HLA C) is widely expressed, being seen on all nucleated cell lineages as a membrane-bound protein and function to expose antigens within the cell to CD8+ cytotoxic T-cells. Class II (HLA DP, HLA DQ, HLA DR), on the other hand, are expressed only within immune lineages and function as presenters of antigen from outside cells to CD4+ T helper cells. A current hypothesis is that MHC molecules expose antigenic portions of drugs as an essential step in how drug allergy arises [69].

2.2.7 History and Physical Examination

Taking a history, doing a physical, and ordering pathology investigations form a key step in assessing the significance of a reaction and deciding whether to diagnose a drug allergy. The past and present drug history, any experience of toxicity, and allergic response to drugs currently or previously used and the relationship in time between exposure and symptomatic presentation, all need to be detailed carefully. All systems with a potential bearing on the clinical presentation need to be included in the physical exam. Skin signs are the way the majority of drug hypersensitivity reactions present. Whilst hypersensitivity reactions can just affect systems other than the skin, the findings then lack specificity and are harder to interpret diagnostically and as a clue to management, thus here skin findings are emphasised for pragmatic reasons. Investigating skin presentations bears significantly on the task of identifying a causative agent, ordering second line tests, and deciding how best to proceed clinically. A large number of skin eruption patterns are found in the literature, such as rashes, hives, angioedema, acne, blistering eruptions, fixed drug eruptions, erythema multiforme, lupus erythematosus, photosensitivity, psoriasis, purpura, vasculitis, itching, and potentially lethal conditions which affect the skin, e.g. Stevens–Johnson syndrome (SJS), toxic epidermal necrolysis (TEN), erythroderma, and drug rash with eosinophilia and systemic symptoms (DRESS) [135].

2.2.8   Diagnostic Tests

A non-exhaustive list of potential investigations encompasses plain chest film, full blood count (including differential), ESR, autoantibodies (nuclear plus cytoplasmic), and specific immunological assays of various kinds. Anaphylaxis may be diagnosed after the event by a positive rise in undifferentiated blood tryptase or active (mature) tryptase. In cases where an allergy to a large molecular weight biologic or penicillin occurring via IgE formation is suspected, the immediate hypersensitivity skin test is of greatest value. A comparatively limited number of studies, with low values for n, have looked at the automated, quantitative assays for IgE and whether they can be applied sufficiently sensitively and specifically to detect IgE to penicillin [136, 137]. Whilst IgE to penicillin is highly specific (97–100%), the test is somewhat less sensitive (29–68%), supplying a high level of confidence that a test positive is a true positive for penicillin drug allergy, but less confidence that a test negative is a true negative.

A newly characterised test which quantifies CD63 levels on basophilic granulocytes following exposure to an allergen is the basophil activation test [138]. Some restricted clinical experience exists about cases of suspected allergic hypersensitivity to β-lactam antibiotics and non-steroidal anti-inflammatory drugs (NSAIDs) where this test has been applied [139–141], but additional comparison with other tests in the market will be required to lead to its being general accepted in diagnostic clinical use. The usual standard for diagnosing contact eczema provoked by topical medications is the patch test, which typically can confirm cases correctly. In the last few years, the literature has contained examples of using patch tests to help diagnose skin eruptions other than those involving IgE, where the drug thought to be responsible has been given systemically [142]. A subset of skin eruptions linked to drugs, which takes in maculopapular rashes, acute generalised exanthematous pustulosis, and fixed drug eruptions can be usefully diagnosed with patch tests [143–145], but otherwise, for SJS and hives, it has no particular value [143–

146]. If several drugs are potentially implicated and the timing between use and hypersensitive reaction remains unclear, dermatopathological biopsy may be of assistance in clarifying if features of a drug eruption are present. Nonetheless, dermatopathological criteria for a drug eruption lack specificity and may not allow other causes to be ruled out [147].

2.2.9 Specific Drugs and Biologic Agents and Drug Allergy

Drug allergies have been found to virtually the entire range of pharmaceuticals, but there are associations of greater occurrence between particular drugs and class of allergic response [84].

2.2.9.1 Antimicrobials

Amongst agents that can provoke an immediate allergic reaction, antibiotics, above all β-lactams, are of prime significance, with around 1 in 10 patients claiming a penicillin allergy. Of these claims, 90% can in fact safely use penicillin, and the label has been misapplied [148, 149]. Substituting broad-spectrum agents to avoid a penicillin allergic response leads to increased costs, compounding of the bacterial resistance issue and can get in the way of providing the highest quality clinical care [150]. If an IgE-facilitated allergic response is suspected, the most dependable method of confirmation is skin testing. The skin testing subset for penicillin allergy (penicilloyl polylysine and penicillin G [151, 152]) has a true negative rate very similar to that of the complete set containing determinants both minor and major [148, 149]. The percentage of patients allergic to penicillin who also respond to cephalosporins has been variously reported. The majority of those with a past penicillin allergy can use cephalosporins [153]; however, on rare occasions anaphylaxis has resulted, with an associated mortality [154]. If a patient has a documented penicillin allergy but tests negatively for the full penicillin skin test set, it is safe to try a cephalosporin [155]. Unlike with the penicillins, there is no standard method for testing cephalosporins or other β-lactams via the skin. Penicillin allergy does not influence allergy rates to monobactams, and the association between penicillin allergy and carbapenems is weak [156, 157]. Whilst IgE may facilitate a reaction to antibiotics outside the β-lactam group, such events are not as frequent as with β-lactams, and in fact, no standard test exists allowing assessment of immediate allergy to such antibiotics [84].

2.2.9.2   Insulin and Oral Antidiabetic Drugs

There have been few reports of allergy following on the use of purified human recombinant insulin, and its prevalence in patients is below 1% [158–161], but amongst those reports have been potentially lethal responses to both insulin and its analogues (aspart, lispro, and glargine). Confirmation of the diagnosis can be made by within-skin testing and/or by serological investigation [162, 163]. How the immune system reacts to recombinant insulin is currently obscure, but aggregation-aligned misfolding has been hypothesised to be responsible [164].

2.2.9.3   Cancer Chemotherapeutic Agents

An allergic response has been noted to almost the entire range of frequently encountered chemotherapy agents, covering a spectrum from skin eruptions at the mild end to severe and fatal anaphylaxis. The antigenic portion may be an excipient, e.g. Kolliphor-EL, used to dissolve a range of chemotherapeutic compounds for intravenous usage, such as paclitaxel, rather than the active agent itself. Up to 42% of patients receiving their first dose of the taxanes, paclitaxel, and docetaxel respond anaphylactically [165], which points to a probable anayphylactoid mechanism. Administering corticosteroids and histamine blockers systemically in advance counters the response in greater than

90% of cases [166]; moreover, of those for whom this precaution fails, desensitisation normally can be induced [167–169].

A different way of managing reactions to paclitaxel is substituting docetaxel, which is generally better tolerated [170]. It is a characteristic of chemotherapeutic agents containing platinum that they induce allergic reactions following multiple courses of treatment [171, 172], a fact which points towards some effect upon the immune system. Administration of prophylactic steroid and histamine blocker does not stop these reactions from occurring [173]. It has been discovered that applying undiluted agent cutaneously can single out patients likely to react allergically, and repetition of this procedure is recommended prior to each set of administrations [172, 174, 175]. A number of schemes to desensitise patients rapidly to the drugs have been described, but with variable rates of success [172, 174, 175]. A newly reported trial of a desensitisation scheme, involving 12 sequential actions to be taken, claimed a success rate of 100% across 413 drug courses of chemotherapy (including platinum compounds) and 94% of these resulted in at most a mild response, often no response at all [169].

2.2.9.4   Medications for Patients with HIV Infections and AIDS

Allergies to drugs are frequently observed in HIV-positive patients, and on occasion, there is an association between frequency of reaction and immunological dysfunction [176–180]. The treatment of AIDS-associated pneumonia caused by *Pneumocystis jirovecii* is rendered more difficult, and the outlook worsens when an allergy to sulphonamides occurs, in most cases in the form of a measles-like, maculopapular rash coincident with pyrexia and appearing 7–12 days into treatment. There are multiple varying procedures known to be successful in desensitising patients with HIV who have had a characteristic maculopapular exanthem appear after taking trimethoprim and sulphamethoxazole [181–192]. The mechanism responsible for changing the immune reaction to trimethoprim-sulphamethoxa-

zole in desensitisation protocols is unknown, as is the scale of
the change. A study of RCT design comparing drug desensitisation with single dosage rechallenge found that the two options
succeeded about equally well (79% and 72%), with no statistical
difference between groups [149]. Procedures to desensitise
allergic AIDS patients to sulphadiazine, acyclovir, zidovudine,
dapsone, and pentamidine also exist [193–198].

2.2.9.5 Medications for Autoimmune Diseases

Gold salts, D-penicillamine, sulphasalazine, hydroxychloro-
quine, and leflunomide, which are all DMARDS (disease-modifying antirheumatic drugs) may each provoke immune reactions,
including DRESS syndrome, light-sensitive dermatitis, toxic
epidermal necrolysis, and vasculitis.

There are now more recently introduced immune-modifying
drugs in the market for a number of autoimmune conditions.
Whilst allergic responses have been documented for these, the
picture is not yet sufficiently complete to evaluate how much of
an impact ADRs may produce worldwide on various immune
control strategies at an early stage of development. Long-
standing skin conditions treated with immunosuppressants and
anti-inflammatories may also be complicated by allergic reactions to these agents. Alongside ADRs that are pharmacologi-
cally based, idiosyncratic (allergic) reactions are on record for
macrolides (such as cyclosporine, tacrolimus, pimecrolimus,
and sirolimus), dapsone, and mycophenolate mofetil, drugs used
by dermatologists to suppress immune function [84].

2.2.9.6 Perioperative Agents and Blood Products

During administration of a general anaesthetic, either anaphylaxis or anaphylactoid responses may occur, attributable to
agents used in induction, neuromuscular blockers, antimicrobi-

als, opiate analgesia, and latex rubber. Due to the inability to differentiate between anaphylaxis and anaphylactoid (extra-immune) responses, experts recommend serum levels of histamine, tryptase, and IgE titres (where possible) be taken at the time, with dermal testing to follow later [199]. Protamine is documented as having led to immediate systemic responses such as hypotension, circulatory collapse, and mortality [200, 201]. Insulin that contains protamine conveys a 40- to 50-fold enhanced risk of anaphylaxis in diabetics [202, 203].

Transfusions of blood and blood-derived products may provoke hives, anaphylactic reactions (even more so if the patient is totally deficient in IgA), anaphylactoid responses, and TRALI (transfusion-related acute lung injury), a syndrome of high complexity giving symptoms and signs in many organ systems which has newly been recognised as a significant contributor to morbidity and death following transfusions [84, 204, 205].

2.2.9.7   Opiates

Opiates and derived compounds frequently lead to pseudoallergy, with symptoms usually being mild and not potentially lethal. Pseudoallergy can be countered by providing H1 antagonists prophylactically. Evaluating cutaneous tests for opiate allergy is complicated by the fact that opiates themselves always trigger histamine release by dermal mast cells [84].

2.2.9.8   Corticosteroids

The usual allergic reaction to corticosteroids is eczema following topical usage. Immediate-type allergic responses do occur, but seldomly, the majority of such reactions documented being in the context of intravenously administered methylprednisolone and hydrocortisone [206–211]. Substances added to prolong shelf life and for dilution may also be responsible [84].

2.2.9.9   Heparin

Hypersensitivity following administration of low molecular weight heparin or unfractionated heparin is rare but may result in low platelet counts, rashes of different kinds, raised circulating eosinophils, and anaphylactic reactions. Slight thrombocytopenia may in fact result from platelets clumping together, and this is the case for 1–3% of patients on unfractionated heparin. When severe, though, thrombocytopenia arises due to immune complexation, partially attributable to IgG targeting platelet factor IV [212]. In this case, it happens for the most part following approximately 5 days' unfractionated heparin administration and thrombosis and necrosis are also observed. A spike in anaphylaxis following heparin observed in Germany and the USA in recent times seems to have been due to a contaminant in the form of an oversulphated chondroitin sulphate compound. The contaminant demonstrably causes the kinin–kallikrein pathway to become active both in humans and in the laboratory. As a result, levels of bradykinin (a powerful modulator of vascular function) rise, alongside C3a and C5a complement peptides [213].

2.2.9.10   Local Anaesthetics

The majority of ADRs linked to local anaesthetic agents operate not through IgE, but some other non-immune mechanism, such as vasovagal reflexes, anxiety, responses linked to toxicity, such as cardiac dysrhythmias, plus reactions of a toxic or idiosyncratic nature attributable to accidentally introducing epinephrine into a blood vessel. It is only very seldom that one encounters a report showing the involvement of IgE [214–217]. Supposing an allergy has previously been documented, testing on the skin and challenging step-by-step seem defensible steps to take to assess the situation [84].

2.2.9.11 Radio-Contrast Media

Anaphylactoid responses are triggered in around 1–3% of recipients of ionic radio-contrast media (RCM), but below 1 in 200 of those receiving non-ionic agents [218, 219]. Potentially lethal, extreme responses occur with less frequency, for ionic RCM in 0.22% of cases, for non-ionic RCM in 0.04% [220]. Being female, asthmatic or having had an earlier anaphylactoid reaction to different RCM all increase the risk of a new anaphylactoid response, whilst taking a beta-blocker plus/minus a comorbid cardiovascular disorder elevates the risk of a more serious anaphylactoid response occurring [221–225].

A range of allergic responses are caused by aspirin and NSAIDs, such as the worsening of pre-existing respiratory disorders, hives, angioedema, anaphylaxis, and from time-to-time pneumonitis and meningitis. AERD is a syndrome wherein aspirin or NSAIDs provoke respiratory responses in patients who suffer from chronic rhinosinusitis or are asthmatic, but its place in the classification scheme for ADRs is unclear. AERD occurs through a pathological alteration of arachidonic acid metabolism. The cysteinyl leukotriene 1 receptor expression is upgraded within the respiratory system, and inhaled leukotriene E4 gives an amplified response [226, 227]. If the patient uses aspirin, the cyclooxygenase 1 enzyme (COX-1) is inhibited, causing a fall in prostaglandin E2 levels. Since the physiological function of prostaglandin E2 is to decrease 5-lipoxygenase activity, a fall in the former leads to enhanced 5-lipoxygenase activity and increased conversion of arachidonic acid to cysteinyl leukotrienes. NSAIDs with a higher affinity for COX-2 than COX-1 will still bind to COX-1 above a certain dose and thus may trigger an AERD response. However, COX-2-specific agents very seldom trigger such problems and thus are generally safe to use in cases of known AERD [228–232].

2.2.9.12   Biologic Modifiers

There have been reports of allergies arising from the use of cytokines, amongst which the interferons and anti-tumour necrosis
factor alpha (TNF-α) are implicated. Recombinant interferons
provoke symptoms ranging from skin eruptions to life-threatening anaphylaxis. In the treatment of both adult and juvenile
forms of rheumatoid arthritis, Crohn's disease, and psoriasis,
infliximab (Remicade) treatment has led to several immunological responses, amongst which the following have been reported:
hives, exacerbation of eczema, maculopapular exanthemata,
hypersensitivity vasculitis, serum sickness and, on a minimum
of seven occasions, anaphylaxis at a severity where life may be
lost. Adalimumab (Humira) is a recently licensed anti-TNF-α
monoclonal antibody, with protein sequence harmonised to naturally occurring human antibodies, which seems to provoke
fewer ADRs, these being confined to itch and rash around the
site of injection and asthma provocation where no previous history existed [84].

2.3   Venom Allergy

2.3.1   Background

Anaphylaxis may be defined as a type of allergic response that
may result in death. Foodstuffs, drugs, and insects are the three
top causes of anaphylaxis. Whilst each of the top three causes
are responsible for a great deal of suffering and deaths, insect
allergy alone can be countered by ways other than the strict
avoidance of contact with antigen. Given that allergy to insects
is linked to more than 40 deaths annually, it is paramount for
clinicians and the general public to know how to recognise the
condition and be aware of how it, as a potentially lethal condition, may be treated in the long term. In contrast with allergies to
foodstuffs and drugs, the management of which relies heavily on
keeping away from triggers, allergy to the order *Hymenoptera*

can be treated proactively through venom immunotherapeutic interventions. Approaching 98% of sufferers can be protected by this means [233].

The insect order Hymenoptera has as members ants, bees, wasps, hornets, and yellow jackets, and these collectively cause most of the lethal or near-lethal incidents involving stings. A knowledge of the ecology and behaviour of hymenopteridae may assist with advising patients on how to avoid contact. An insect allergy diagnosis depends upon an account of a whole body reaction consistent with allergy following a sting and serological confirmation of IgE to insect venom. Where these criteria for diagnosis are met, venom immunotherapeutics should be used. Acute episodes of anaphylaxis, though, necessitate administration of epinephrine without delay: research reveals that emergency practice falls short of this recommendation [233].

The class Insecta (which covers the insects) is part of the Arthropod phylum. Developmentally, mature adult organisms possess a rigid exoskeleton, anatomically divided by three into head, thorax, and abdomen segments and paired, jointed legs, six legs in total. As a class, Insecta are the most varied and plentiful of the Kingdom Animalia. Amongst this variety, we find the multiple types of mantis, dragonflies, grasshoppers, true bugs, flies, flees, bees, wasps, ants, lice, butterflies, moths, and beetles, with an estimated total species count somewhere around six to ten million, of which one million have been scientifically catalogued to date. At least half of all living creatures currently known to exist are insects, but the true contribution of insects to the biodiversity of the planet may be even more than 90%. Clearly, no human can escape meeting with insects, but the levels of contact with those insects (or body parts thereof) that do bite or sting can go from the scarcely appreciable to lethal levels of contact [234].

The stinger itself generally takes the form of a pointed organ for attack or defence, frequently coupled with a venomous gland, which functions through penetrative injury to the victim, such as occurs with a scorpion's tail sting. Anatomically, it is mostly found in the posterior portion of the insect. Some insects equipped for stinging include bees, wasps, hornets, and scorpions [234].

The majority of the insects which sting are Hymenopteridae [235], an order which contains numerous families, of which three have medical significance: bees (apid family), wasps (vespid family), and ants (formicid family). Bee stings have barbs and the sting breaks off the bee's body, entailing death for the animal after stinging even once. Since the stings of Vespidae (wasps, hornets, and yellowjackets) are unbarbed, they can sting repeatedly [236]. Fire ants frequently change position and reattach themselves to a victim to facilitate repeated stings, the effect of which is to make the victim feel the stung area is on fire. Fire ants may gather in a large group and then fix onto a victim before releasing their stings all at once, an effect triggered by an alarm pheromone originating from one or several ants. Such an attack can be severe and produce pustulation due to formic acid being forced into the skin. Older persons or those with limited mobility risk being enveloped in a swarm of ants, the attack being of a severity that can be life-threatening [234].

Stings from apidae and vespidae are non-identical, and the principal allergenic compounds of both have been carefully isolated. Whilst these two categories of stings share a hyaluronidase component, only bees secrete phospholipase A2 and mellitin, and only wasps secrete antigen 5. There is little crossreactivity between bee and wasp stings [237]. Wasp stings are infrequent, occurring possibly a single time every decade or 15 years, provided the patient's job does not entail a greater risk [237].

The outstanding emergency risk from coming into contact with insects relates to anaphylaxis. Insect saliva, venom, body parts, excretion, or secretory products may be innocuous to many, but, where allergy occurs, may cause a whole body reaction. Prompt recognition of whole body allergic signs and symptoms that presage anaphylaxis is essential to manage cases where contact with insects is thought to have taken place, since anaphylaxis can claim lives even in a 10 min window following the emergence of symptoms [234].

There is a risk of between 40 and 60% that a sting suffered later will again provoke anaphylaxis. Tell the patient how to avoid potential contact with the allergen and supply an epinephrine auto-injector, with training on appropriate usage, whenever the risk of a future anaphylactic reaction is considered significant [238].

2.3.2   Pathophysiology

There are three ways insects use their mouthparts to bite: they may pierce the skin, employ sponging, or a straight bite. The anatomy of biting insects is highly varied. Whilst the majority of the insects mentioned here lack venom, a great deal of species transfer saliva to the wound when they do bite. The function of the saliva may be to assist with digesting food, prevent cessation of blood flow to the area, or prevent the victim perceiving the bite. The majority of pathological responses to bites are immune-mediated. Chagas' disease occurs when the microorganism responsible (found within reduviid frass) has been inadvertently introduced into the wound by the victim following itching and scratching of the bite area. The majority of bites are not serious and may simply cause slight dermal injury from puncture. The horsefly may inflict a more penetrating and tender injury due to its biting mechanism: a proboscis that resembles a pair of shears [234].

There are numerous protein components within venoms capable of eliciting an allergic response; mostly they are enzymes. Whilst honeybees produce toxins which can be distinguished molecularly from those produced by other Hymenopteridae, the wasps' stings are virtually identical from an allergenic standpoint, with corresponding cross-reactive potential. If a patient has an allergy to wasps, in the majority of cases, the skin tests will be positive for the full set of yellow jacket, yellow hornet, and white-faced hornet. Amongst vespidae, the Polistes genus is distinct, and thus cross-reactivity between yellow jacket allergy and paper wasp allergens is no more than 50%.

By contrast, the fire ant sting contains only low levels of proteinaceous material within a solution of alkaloid toxins. These alkaloids are responsible for the vesicle formation that is typically the fire ant sting response in victims. There is no cross-reactivity between wasp and fire ant sting proteins except in a single case that explains the limited cross-reaction. Materials for diagnosis and treatment sold currently are made from whole fire ants. The extracts so prepared are better suited to stimulate response in skin testing than comparable ones made from other whole insects and are of greater use in prophylactic immune treatments [239, 240].

2.3.3   Epidemiology

Allergy to hymenopterid toxins is defined as an allergic response to the sting or stings of bees, wasps, polistes wasps, hornets, or fire ants, which may occasion death. Adults exceed children for the risk of an anaphylactic response to hymenopterid stings, attributable to the presence of other simultaneous conditions and the prevalence of medicines reliance in this age bracket. Reports reveal a prevalence of 3% amongst adults, but only 0.34% amongst children [241–243].

In 2014, some 30,738 instances in which an individual was stung by an insect were noted by the American Association of Poison Control Centers (AAPCC) [244], of which slightly over 1500 produced a moderate, and somewhat under 40 a major, response. Moderate refers to clearly noticeable or whole body effects, whilst major refers to potential lethality or leaving the patient with disabling problems. It should be emphasised that underreporting to the American Poison Centres makes these figures artefactually lower than the true incidence. Deaths caused by insects are seldom notified to poison centres. They usually arise from a hymenopterid allergy. Thus the official figures give only a tentative indication of the true level [244].

Allergies to stinging insects happen at all ages, preceded in many cases by several stings that caused no special problem. They used to be reckoned less common than they are now. About 3% of adults state they have had a whole body allergic response to a sting, whilst severe responses in children are reported in just under 1% [245, 246]. Whilst the incidence of large local reaction remains debateable, a figure of 10% has been proposed. In the USA on an annual basis, 50 or more stings result in an allergic response that ends in death [247], and half the time these deaths occur with no evidence of responding allergically to a previous sting. Indeed, death due to sting may be frequently overlooked as an explanation. In a number of cases where blood was taken at autopsy, venom serology for IgE and a high tryptase result have led to a putative diagnosis of fatal sting response where otherwise the death cannot be accounted for [248, 249]. Nonetheless, IgE to hymenopterid toxins can be normal and is fairly common. In cases where an adult had sustained a sting within the previous 3 months, IgE to venom was detectable by skin test or RAST in 30%, whilst above 20% of adults showed a test positive to yellow jacket or honeybee toxins, despite never having had any symptoms of allergy to stings [245]. In these asymptomatic individuals, the sensitivity is temporary, lasting less time than in individuals who have experienced anaphylaxis. 30–60% of cases with a test positive (skin) were test negative some 3–6 years later. Those for whom the test kept on showing positive had whole body reactions to stings on 17% of occasions [250].

2.3.4   Symptoms

There is a range of symptoms that can occur: large local reactions are at the site of injury; whole body reactions range from mild to severe. "Mild" whole body reactions are represented principally by cutaneous responses including flushing, hives, and angioedema. "Moderate" essentially refers to lightheadedness, difficulty breathing, and feeling like vomiting. "Severe" encompasses anaphylactic shock, asthma, loss of consciousness and arrest (cardiac or respiratory). Life quality is worsened greatly by being afraid that another such event may occur in the future. Approximately 25% of deaths caused by anaphylaxis are linked to insect venoms [110, 251, 252].

In the absence of a specific allergy, being stung by bees or wasps leads to severe pain at the area of injury, erythematous reaction occurring immediately and an oedematous reaction of 1 cm or less diameter at the site. Allergic responses may be localised or systemic [234, 237].

2.3.4.1 Local Reactions

Oedema surrounding the puncture site accompanies local reactions, developing in hours and of variable extent, potentially, though, over a whole hand or complete limb. Blisters may form in dependent areas, and an infection may develop. Provided the airway is not compromised, oedema is not in itself a cause for concern [237].

2.3.4.2 Generalised Reactions

Generalised (whole body) reactions exhibit a high degree of heterogeneity with regard to severity. Redness of the skin and itching are amongst the first signs, after which hives and angioedema of the face or elsewhere may occur. It is not unusual for someone undergoing extreme systemic reactions to have a profound sense of being unwell, with *angor animi* ("sense of impending doom"). Difficulty drawing breath is frequently concomitant as a consequence of either swelling of the larynx or asthmatic responses. Blood pressure drops markedly during extreme reactions, occasioning dizziness, unsteadiness, swooning or passing out. Abdominodynia, loss of urinary control, retrosternal pain, or changes to vision are more unusual accompaniments [237].

How patients present differs considerably: cutaneous lesions such as reddening of the skin, hives, and angioedema may occur as a complete picture; but, equally, obtundation may rapidly supervene following a vague initial presentation, even minutes after receiving venom. Systemic reactions occur speedily, the time frame typically being less than 10 min post injury [237].

It is advisable that patients have a resuscitation package on their person, with H1 blockers, steroids and epinephrine auto-injector, as indicated by earlier responses to stinging. The sole therapeutic modality with the hope of thwarting recurrence of extreme responses is venom immunotherapy (VIT), which potentially confers clinical benefits over a prolonged period and supplies a greater life quality [253, 254]. Despite this, VIT is less utilised by either doctors or patients than would be expected [243, 255].

2.3.5 Diagnosis

To diagnose an allergy to insect venom, a plausible account together with IgE serology (looking for venom antibodies) is required. The degree to which the patient has correctly identified the stinging animal needs to be taken into account, as many wasp stings are incorrectly attributed to bees by victims. In fact, allergies are usually due to vespid venom, unless exceptional exposure (e.g. beekeeping) has occurred. Diagnosis informs therapy, hence its importance [237].

It is regrettable that cutaneous testing is not beneficial for screening and thus only indicated where a generalised allergic response has happened following the patient being stung. If patients could be screened for an allergy to insects in advance of the first sting, such a procedure might stop deaths and disability resulting from a first anaphylactic response, but currently, one in two of mortalities attributable to stings has had no herald event preceding them. VIT cannot be given on the basis of positive skin tests alone, given that tests frequently indicate positivity in adults who have had exposure to stings but have not developed any hypersensitivity. It should be reserved for where generalised reactions have already occurred. Theoretically, immunoglobulin

E to venom cannot be produced without an event of exposure, but some reports of unprovoked hypersensitivity have been documented. Clinical experience suggests that a collateral history encompassing early childhood exposure often reveals an exposure event not remembered by the patient [245]. An alternative hypothesis is that plant allergens (pollen inhaled or foodstuffs) induce cross-reactions or that the epitope is a carbohydrate rather than protein [256, 257].

Cutaneous testing for venom allergy is the most popular option for diagnosis thanks to being both highly sensitive and associated with low clinical risk [258], whilst laboratory investigations lack sensitivity and may provide false reassurance. The test has been standardised by using an extract of venom from five families of hymenopterids, and whole fire ant extract. These antigens are introduced intradermally, at a concentration of between 0.001 and 1.0 µg/mL, titrating upwards until a positive result is elicited. Those who have previously had markedly extreme allergic responses may be tested initially at less than 1 µL per mL concentration. A sufferer may have cross-reactivity to many different stings despite only having responded to one species, hence the use of the five families' extract. Simultaneously with the antigenic extract, a negative control with HSA-saline plus positive histamine-only control should be tested [239].

Between 65 and 85% of patients who describe convincingly an allergic response to stings do in fact have a positive skin test. Of the negative tests, some are accounted for by downgraded hypersensitivity after a prolonged period, whilst in others who have had an anaphylactic response to stings, an anergic interlude may last some weeks following the reaction. In the latter case, repetition of the test between 1 and 6 months later is advisable [259].

A different option is to quantify IgE specific to the various venoms through a radioallergosorbent test (RAST) or the various newer assay methods now available [237]. One such technique with an improved detection rate is CAP-RAST. The technique is reported to have a false-positive rate (here defined as IgE positivity to vespid and apid venom, when truly positive to only one type) of approaching 30%. The RAST by comparison has a false-positivity rate of 6%, too. Allergy is a clinical diagnosis that does not correspond exactly to the existence of specific immunoglobulin, but lacking clinical features, which may be better termed sensitisation. Seldom is a patient allergic to both vespid and apid venom. Unless the history can be confirmed, and IgE levels for apid- and vespid-specific venom checked, misdiagnosis can occur. Population studies reveal instances where an individual has been stung, has produced corresponding IgE, but has shown no clinical features of hypersensitivity [237].

2.3.6 Prognosis

Aside from the categories of extreme anaphylaxis where medical intervention fails to occur, and superimposed invasive or persistent infections, the prognosis is favourable overall [234]. Deaths that happen following insect stings are caused by three factors: anaphylaxis (IgE mediated), anaphylactoid (not through IgE), or infectious sequelae. According to the American Centers for Disease Control and Prevention, anaphylaxis following stings accounts for an estimated 90–100 deaths per annum [260]. Anaphylaxis due to insects is worse in patients who are elderly, already have a cardiovascular disorder or disease affecting mast cells, are on treatment with beta-blockers or ACE inhibitors, and who have had an extreme hypersensitivity response before. Honeybee stings are more dangerous than other types [261].

Local reactions cause the following patient complaints: discomfort, pruritus, moderate or marked aching, skin redness, area painful to touch, warmth, and oedematous surrounding skin. Whilst joints may be affected in a local reaction, generalised symptoms should be absent. If the local reaction is extreme, there may be widespread skin redness, hives, and swelling caused by scratching. A marked local reaction may herald a future generalised response, following re-exposure to a sting.

A generalised, anaphylaxis response may consist of a mixture of localised, as well as anatomically distant, signs and symptoms, from mild symptoms to actual death. Symptoms that develop first are widespread exanthems, hives, itching, and angioedema, but these may develop further into a feeling of dread, being disorientated, debility, gut symptoms (griping, loose stools, vomiting), cramp from the uterus in females, loss of bowel or bladder control, lightheadedness, fainting, drop in blood pressure, noisy breathing, difficulty breathing, or coughing. Anaphylaxis may lead to respiratory collapse and cardiovascular insufficiency [262].

Postponed responses emerge 10–14 days post stinging event. They present similarly to those in serum sickness, with pyrexia, malaise, headache, hives, swelling of lymph glands, and arthritic pain in several joints at once [234].

2.3.7   Treatment

If a local reaction extends over a wide area, oedema can be reduced using ice compresses. The maximal duration for which ice can be applied is quarter of an hour, and a cloth should be interposed between ice and flesh to avoid thermal injury occurring. In generalised responses, the most important thing before taking the patient to hospital is to administer epinephrine, by whichever route (subcutaneous, intramuscular, into a vein, via the trachea) is most suitable in view of the skill level of the person administering the drug and the clinical condition of the patient. Systemic histamine blockade and steroidal administration are of benefit in generalised reactions. It is common for sufferers of bee sting allergy to keep with them a set of materials for use after a sting. An epinephrine auto-injector is included. See also section on hymenopterid stings [234].

Antihistamines for topical use are unsuitable for extensive area coverage and are to be avoided if systemic H1 blockade is being administered. Using antihistamines inappropriately can produce toxic effects via the widespread cholinergic system. It is, however, acceptable to use H1 and H2 blockers together (H2 being used for gastric acid overproduction). For many cases, going to hospital will not be required, but it is needed if a generalised response is apparent or if insects have caused an anaphylactic reaction before. Telephone advice from a regional poison centre can help eliminate expensive and unnecessary attendance at Accident and Emergency [234].

A more in-depth discussion of hymeopterid stings is under that section, but it is worth noting that bee stings that remain in situ necessitate removal. Whilst it was previously advised that stings be removed by a scraping action, thus preventing inadvertent expulsion of the remaining venom in the gland into the skin, it is now known that the gland automatically contracts even after removal from the bee itself and thus the venom is usually all emptied very quickly. What matters is to get rid of the sting; how that happens is unimportant [234].

2.3.7.1   Emergency Department Care

It may be necessary to intubate and ventilate patients with severe anaphylaxis or where the airway is compromised through angioedema [234].

A patient with an allergic diathesis who appears to be developing anaphylaxis can first be given an injection of 0.3–0.5 mL of 1:1000 epinephrine into a muscle, with the option to repeat each 10 min if required. Anaphylaxis from an insect bite is far rarer than from stings. See also section on hymenoterid stings [234].

If a case of anaphylaxis is extreme, intravenous administration of epinephrine (1:10,000) (usually within 10 mL vials) may be contemplated, but with caution. A satisfactory strategy at the beginning is to give several 1 mL boluses intravenously if anaphylaxis has led to a critical clinical condition. When the patient begins to recover following these 1 mL administrations, they can be replaced by continuous epinephrine intravenous infusion, under close supervision. To eliminate the danger of accidentally overdosing the patient on intravenous epinephrine, careful attention should be paid to concentration, dosage, and form being administered [234].

Since cases with extremely low blood pressure are often managed with extensive intravenous fluids, it is essential to check the level of angioedema and retained fluid in the lungs [234].

Both H1 and H2 blockade can be of help to treat a generalised reaction. Accident and Emergency suites generally employ diphenhydramine; however, a useful alternative, unless intravenous administration is required, is cetirizine, which has equal efficacy, comparable onset of effect and lasts longer. Steroids are used as a matter of course in such cases [234].

Tetanus immunisation should also be undertaken, if not already done [234].

Skin redness that lacks a clear limit and with accompanying oedema may mimic cellulitis. Given that infection only occurs in less than 50% of cases, treating blindly with antibiotics is not advised [234].

Epinephrine (Adrenalin, Bronitin, EpiPen)

Epinephrine is the first and best first step in treating shock, angioedema, compromised airway, spasm of the bronchi, and hives in extreme anaphylaxis. It is normally given intramuscularly, but, if a patient is about to die, intravenously. If venous access is problematic, sublingual or endotracheal routes can be used. If shock does not respond to bolus injection, a non-stop infusion can be set up [234].

Bronchodilators

β-Agonists activate an intramembrane ATPase which responds to cAMP (cyclic adenosine monophoshate), which then shuttles potassium intracellularly to produce an adrenergic action [234].

Salbutamol (Ventolin)

Salbutamol can be employed to release bronchial spasm that has not responded to epinephrine. It is a beta-2 agonist, which acts on smooth muscle without affecting cardiac muscle or heart function. Salbutamol is the most frequently used bronchodilator for alleviation of bronchial spasm, but there are a number of other inhaled beta-agonists with comparable pharmacology [234].

Antihistamines

The effect of histaminergic release in the allergic symptomatic response can be countered by any of multiple H1 antagonists. An effective and easily obtained agent is diphenhydramine [234].

Where an H1 antagonist on its own has not remedied pruritus and flushing from anaphylaxis, or itching, hives and contact eczema, an H2 blocker can be used in addition. Cimetidine is recommended [234].

Systemic Corticosteroids

Steroids are anti-inflammatory in action and occasion far-reaching metabolic changes, as well as modulating how the immune system responds to a number of different challenges. Two representatives of the group are prednisolone and its methylated version. The amount reaching the bloodstream is comparable from both parenteral and oral administration. Provided a patient is not about to die, and can swallow easily, give the drug by mouth. If the situation mandates it, however, steroids can be given parenterally [234].

Anti-tetanus Immunoglobulin

Anti-tetanus immunoglobulin confers passive immunity for patients with injuries that may have exposed them to tetanus spores [234].

2.3.7.2 Desensitisation (Immunotherapy)

For a patient who has experienced a systemic reaction, the decision whether to proceed with desensitisation hinges upon the degree of reaction: severe response generally should be desensitised, mild response does not need to be, and moderate reactions may fall into either category. Other aspects to be considered include the likelihood of stings occurring again, the length of time since last stung, comorbidities, how adept the patient may be at self-administration of therapy, and how readily available medical assistance is [262]. Whilst venom immunotherapy has a high level of effectiveness, many venom allergies will resolve without intervention, and treatment has a corresponding adverse event profile which needs to be borne in mind. Approximately 1 in 10 administrations of venom immunotherapy produce a generalised allergic response, and this can include anaphylaxis. Thus, only where adequate expertise and ongoing experience exist should the therapy be undertaken [237].

There are several ways to administer venom immunotherapy. The standard (conventional) regime begins with injections of low venom which are titrated upwards over a 3-month period at weekly intervals. After 3 months, the peak dose of 100 µg is reached, which equates to two stings. Following this, patients need to continue at this dosage for 3 years, the dose being given each month or at a lower frequency [237].

A minimum period of 1 year giving the dose at 4 week intervals is needed. The majority of specialists are in agreement that doses can then be spaced out to 6- or 8-week intervals and given for a number of years.

Cutaneous testing or RAST is performed repeatedly, generally once each 2 or 3 years, with the aim of assessing if venom-specific IgE levels have dropped significantly [263]. Normally, for the initial 2–3 years, cutaneous tests retain positivity, but 4–6 years later, the positivity falls appreciably. After 5 years, under 20% of cases show definite cutaneous test negativity; however, 2–5 years afterwards, between 50 and 60% test negatively, albeit the RAST continues to be positive [264, 265].

Mechanism of immunotherapy

T-cells are responsible for cytokine signalling, whereby the immune system is co-ordinated. T-helper cells may be subdivided into distinct populations (Th1 and Th2) by observing which cytokines they secrete when challenged antigenically [237].

Venom immunotherapy has been demonstrated to produce major differences in the way cytokines are released, favouring the Th1 response over a pathological Th2 pattern. The explanation may be that the pathway via Th2 becomes downgraded (anergy) or that the Th1 pathway becomes more dominant. A combined explanation is also plausible. Th2 cells secrete the proallergic cytokines IL4, IL5, and IL3 (IL = interleukin). IL4 promotes immunoglobulin E production, IL5 activates eosinophils, IL3 mast cells, and both work as chemotactic agents. Venom immunotherapy results in Th2 cells no longer producing cytokines when presented with a venom antigen. Rather, Th1 cells predominate, producing IL2 and interferon gamma, (INF-γ). INF-γ antagonises IL4, preventing B cells switching to IgE production and release. The alteration in cytokine secretions can account for how IgE ceases being produced over the long term, but why desensitisation precedes this phenomenon is mysterious. It would appear that a further mechanism, coming into place earlier, remains to be discovered [237].

2.4 Allergic Rhinitis, Asthma, and Anaphylaxis

2.4.1 Background

One thing that asthma, hay fever, and allergic dermatitis have in common is the involvement of the Th2 subpopulation of T-helper cells, with interleukins 3, 4, and 5 plus 13 being produced, as well as GM-CSF, when exposure to allergens occurs. The pathophysiology features eosinophil-mediated inflammatory responses and a variable amount of mast cell involvement. Disease of greater duration leads to the distortion of the healthy tissue architecture and replacement by regenerated tissues. The organ most affected may depend on where the allergen first provoked hypersensitivity, where ongoing contact occurs, the organ homing predilection of the T-cells and the response pattern of cells at each site [266].

2.4.2 Asthma and Anaphylaxis

In asthma, eosinophils and T-cells invade the small airways as part of an immune response and the smooth muscle of the bronchi constricts. This result is widespread, albeit reversible, airway narrowing. Asthma can be as mild as wheezing occasionally, inability to take a breath properly and coughing at night, or as profoundly severe in causing obstruction of breathing as to endanger life, and covers all stages in between. Amongst the long-term childhood conditions, it has the highest prevalence, with 5–10% of children having the disease. Nine tenths of asthma in children and three tenths of asthma in adults are allergic in type (triggered by some antigen). Specific triggers are found to provoke symptoms, and an allergic diathesis in the patient or relatives is common. House dust mites (*Dermatophagoides pteronyssinus*) or animals, such as cats, provoke symptoms lasting throughout the year (perennial) whilst symptoms tied to particular periods in the year (seasonal) are frequently provoked by pollen hypersensitivity, from trees in March through to May, grasses from June to July and weeds from July to August. Allergic rhinitis and conjunctivitis share many triggers seasonally. Asthma not brought on by exposure to allergens (intrinsic asthma) has the same pathophysiological features, although not dependence on allergenic contact.

A subgroup of asthmatics show sensitivity to aspirin, but the mechanism is not via IgE formation. Being given aspirin or similar drugs lead to markedly extreme closure of airways for sufferers, whilst inflammation of the nose and polyposis secondary to this inflammation is a very frequent finding. Whatever the subtype of asthma, all sufferers have airways that are extremely reactive to irritants that are not acting allergenically, notably viruses, cold air and dust, or pollution in the vicinity [266].

Asthma is a clinical diagnosis, based on the patient's account and any findings from the physical exam that are consistent with the diagnosis (such as wheezing). To verify the diagnosis, peak flow rates should be less than normal on breathing out with maximum effort, but improve when given a bronchodilator. Cutaneous tests or serum total IgE plus IgE titres to common allergens can isolate the allergenic problem. Asthma that is extrinsic has two separate phases, the first of which has its onset less than 30 min after allergenic exposure and is mediated by histamine and other stored chemical signals within mucosally located mast cells that are emitted without delay. The second phase begins some 6–8 h afterwards and is modulated by different signals plus the arrival of lymphocytes and granulocytes. Because the bronchi become hyperactive, patients remains symptomatic for multiple days or weeks following contact with allergen, and this is the key feature of active disease in intrinsic asthma. Steroids delivered by inhalation are the principal way inflammation is countered in asthma, but one should not forget that inhaled bronchodilators have a role, as do anti-inflammatories taken systemically when the severity level is higher. For the majority of cases, desensitisation treatments do not help, and indeed some deaths have occurred when this has been attempted [266].

2.4.2.1 Pathophysiology

The pathological mechanisms underlying asthma are complicated and three elements interact: airways become inflamed, the passage of air through the airways may be obstructed at intervals and the bronchi are hyperreactive. Asthma-associated inflammation can be of an acute, subacute, or chronic form. Oedema within the airways and increased mucous secretions affect the patency of the airways and influence how the bronchi respond. To a greater or lesser extent, the following features occur: mononucleocytosis, eosinophilic invasion, excess mucus production, sloughing off of epithelial surfaces, overgrowth of smooth muscle, and reshaping of the airway [267, 268].

The way the airways, especially the bronchi, respond in patients with asthma is an extreme version of a normal physiological response, brought on by contact with many different internal and external triggers. Airway reactivity works through direct smooth muscle excitation or indirectly via the release of signalling molecules from other cell types, such as mast cells or unmyelinated sensory neurones. There is a strong correlation between how severe the disease is clinically and the amount of extreme response given by the airways [269].

Asthma pathology is a complex subject, but comprises the following factors [269]:

- Inflammation occurring within airways
- Discontinuous blockage of air entry and exit
- Overreactive bronchi

Inflammation Occurring Within Airways

Three subtypes of inflammation coexist in asthmatics: acute, subacute, and chronic. Airflow blockages are produced due to oedematous airways, mucus overproduction, and overreactive bronchi. To a greater or lesser extent, mononucleocytes and eosinophils invade the tissues, mucus is excreted excessively and epithelial layers are sloughed away, smooth muscle proliferates, and airway architecture is changed [268].

Key cellular components involved in inflammation of the airway are mast cells, eosinophils, epitheliocytes, macrophages, and recruited T-cells. T-cells are significant regulators of the inflammation, which they orchestrate through cytokine signalling. The other cells that make up the airway (fibroblasts, cells of the endothelium, and epithelium) influence how chronic the disease becomes. Molecules that regulate cellular adhesion, particularly selectins and integrins, play a central role in modulating the inflammatory response. Cells produce signals that alter smooth muscle tonicity and influence the rearrangement of cellular architecture in the airway [269].

Balzar et al. [270] found that airway mast cell levels differ between the airways of healthy and asthmatic subjects. Increased relative numbers of mast cells expressing chymase and elevated prostaglandin D2 were found to correlate with severe asthma, when levels were compared with those in subjects receiving steroids [269].

Persistent airway inflammation co-occurs with overresponsivity of bronchi, and episodes of spasm of the bronchi are the result, alongside the clinical manifestations of wheezing, being short of breath and cough brought on by contact with the triggers: viruses, allergenic materials, irritating substances, exercising, and cold air.

In cases where persistent disease has remained without treatment for long periods, changes in the airway architecture (hyperplastic and hypertrophic smooth muscle, new vessel formation, and scarring underlying the epithelium) may prevent the full reversal of airway obstruction [269].

The airway-associated inflammation seen in asthma may be a manifestation of disequilibrium between two subpopulations of T-helper cells: Th1 and Th2. Th1 cells modulate whole cell responses to infection via secretion of interleukin 2 (IL2) and IFN-α. Th2 cells, in comparison, modulate allergic responses via production of interleukins 4–6, IL9, and IL13. Gauvreau et al. [271] outlined the function of IL13 in allergenic reactivity of the airways.

A hypothesis which has found much favour recently in explaining why asthma has become more prevalent in Western countries is the "hygiene hypothesis" [272]. According to this explanation, neonatal immune systems have a bias towards Th2-orchestrated responses (i.e. primarily allergic), but this bias is corrected by exposure to infections, etc. in the environment, which lead to greater Th1 activity. Definitive evidence to substantiate this claim is, however, lacking [273].

Discontinuous Blockage of Air Entry and Exit

The contributors to blockage of the airways are acute constriction of bronchi, oedematous airways, persistent plugging by mucus buildup, and airway architectural changes. IgE release following contact with airborne allergens leads to acute bronchoconstriction, the main element in asthma in its early phase.

The accumulated oedema is evident after 6–24 h and is termed the late asthma response. Plugging results from aggregation of plasma proteins with cellular remains and may persist for a number of weeks. The architectural changes to the airway caused by remodelling following persistent inflammation may inhibit attempts to reverse the narrowing [274].

The narrowing of airways hinders the airflow, resulting in a fall in the expiratory flow rate. Since that diminishes the ability to expel air from the lungs, the lungs may become hyperinflated. Whilst this overstretching of lung capacity does beneficially tend to keep the airways open, and thus allow greater airflow on expiration, it does so at the cost of altering lung mechanical function and rendering breathing more laborious [269].

Overreactive Bronchi

Hyperinflating the lungs can only remedy the blockage to airflow up to a certain point, since, if the tidal volume is close to the volume of the anatomical dead space, the alveoli will remain underventilated. The variability in resistance to airflow between different areas of the bronchial tree causes air to be delivered unevenly across the lungs. The air pressure in the alveoli also varies due to the overstretching of the lung, and the uncoupling of ventilation and perfusion results, worsened by the reflex vasoconstriction occurring at the alveolar level due to relatively anaerobic conditions. On some occasions, however, the vasoconstrictive reflex may be beneficial [269].

Whilst an asthma episode is developing, patients may have hypoxia but without the expected hypercarbia. This is due to the ease with which carbon dioxide diffuses across the membranes separating circulatory and air spaces. Hypoxia is a consequence of ventilation-perfusion uncoupling. The arterial carbon dioxide partial pressure also reduces as a result of patients hyperventilating due to the hypoxic drive. Early in an acute episode, the alveolar receives overventilation and this too blocks the formation of hypercarbia. As airway blockage increases and the uncoupled ventilation-perfusion mechanisms become more disequilibriated, carbon dioxide begins to accumulate; hence, hypercarbia will develop. Viewed from a metabolic perspective, the early stages are characterised by alkalosis from low CO_2 levels resulting from hyperventilation, whereas the later stages are characterised by acidosis, a result of the metabolic demands of breathing itself, higher oxygen demand, and the heart pumping harder. As respiratory failure sets in, the alveoli no longer receive sufficient ventilation and the level of retained CO_2 rises even further, resulting in a further tendency to acidosis [269].

2.4.2.2   Aetiology

The following may worsen asthma or the overresponsivity of the airways [269]:

- Allergenic materials from the environment (e.g. house dust mite, cats and dogs (or other animals to a lesser extent), cockroaches, and fungal sources).
- Viruses that affect the respiratory organs.
- Exercise or hyperventilation.
- Acid reflux disease.
- Persistent rhinitis or sinusitis.
- Sensitivity to aspirin, other NSAIDs or sulphites.
- β-Blockers, systemic or topical (such as in ophthalmology).
- Being obese [275].
- Polluted air including from smoking.
- Occupation-linked.
- Irritant exposure (aerosols, paint fumes).
- Assorted chemical triggers, not characterised by molecular size, such as insects, plants, rubber, gums, diisocyanates, anhydrides, dust from woodworking, various flux materials— an example of occupational exposure.
- Psychological factors including response to stressful events.
- Perinatally, mother's age being high, being born prematurely, mother smoking, exposure in utero to tobacco toxins. Breastfeeding cannot be proven beyond doubt to be of benefit.

2.4.2.3   Manifestations of an Acute Episode

Acute asthma is divided clinically as follows: mild, moderate severity, high severity, pre-respiratory arrest [269].

Mild Episodes

Breathlessness may be associated with physical exercise, e.g. walking. Patients can speak in full sentences and are able to lie in bed, although they may feel distressed. Mild asthma does not prevent patients from lying flat. Respiratory rates are higher than usual, but the respiratory accessory muscles do not feature. There is no tachycardia nor *pulsus paradoxus* (systolic fall whilst breathing in). Auscultatory findings show moderate wheeze, commonly at the end of expiration. If no wheezing is present, asking the patient to breathe out forcibly may unmask its presence. Oxygen saturation should be above 95% on air [269].

Moderate Severity

As with mild episodes, an increase in respiratory rate is expected, but now accessory muscles may be employed. In paediatric cases, supraclavicular and intercostal retraction, nostril flaring, and abdominal breathing should be checked for. A tachycardia of approaching 120 bpm is found. Wheezing is audible and loud and *pulsus paradoxus* with 10–20 mmHg difference is observable on occasion. Oxygen saturation on air is between 91 and 95%. Talking triggers breathlessness. Infants cannot feed properly and cry more quietly and for less time than usual. As severity worsens, patients feel the need to sit up [269].

High Severity

The patient experiences breathlessness even at rest, loses appetite, remains sitting upright, uses less than full sentences, and is typically distressed. Respiratory rate may frequently exceed 30 per minute. The accessory muscles are characteristically in use and suprasternal retractions frequently occur. Tachycardia exceeds 120 bpm. Easily audible wheezing occurs whilst both breathing in and breathing out. *Pulsus paradoxus* may be present with a 20–40 mmHg deflection. Oxygen saturation goes below 91%. With progressive decline, the posture becomes bent forward, with hands on knees ("tripod position") [269].

Pre-respiratory Arrest

Young children about to experience respiratory arrest show drowsiness and disorientation as well as the symptoms of high severity, but adolescents may remain alert and oriented up to the point respiratory failure has started. For asthmatics about to arrest, the usual respiratory movements of chest and abdomen are reversed. Wheezing may have disappeared (due to a very high level of airway blockage) and hypoxia of sufficient severity may now result in bradycardia. *Pulsus paradoxus* may also have disappeared, indicative of fatigue in the muscles of respiration [269].

With progressive worsening, sweating may be intense, occurring at the same time as the carbon dioxide rises and respiratory rate declines. For extreme cases, patients may be visibly highly distressed and disorientated, taking off any oxygen supply because they mistakenly feel it is preventing them from breathing. This clinical picture correlates with hypoxia severe enough to cause death. As the patient becomes more hypercapnic, respiratory rate may slow, and they may become drowsy and sweat profusely. Breath sounds may be virtually lost. The patients are content to lie flat [269].

2.4.2.4 Symptoms of an Asthma Emergency

The following are warning signs that asthma is at a level to require emergency intervention [276]:

- Breathlessness at rest
- Difficulty with even slight exertion
- Feeling anxious
- Failure of symptoms to remit following initial inhaler usage

- Recording a peak flow measurement which fails to reach 50% of the patient's best level
- Perioral cyanosis or cyanosis of the fingertips
- Debility or disorientation
- Intercostal retractions (particularly for children)
- Loss of consciousness (LoC)

  Anaphylaxis presents as follows [277]:

- Exanthem
- Oedema, particularly laryngeal
- LoC
- Wheezing, dyspnoea, chest tightness
- Dysphagia
- Dysphonia
- Emesis, diarrhoea, and intestinal colic
- Facial blanching or erythema

2.4.2.5   Incidence of Anaphylactic Shock in Asthma

A cohort study reported an annual occurrence rate for anaphylactic shock of 19.9 per 100,000 people-years in a control group, but 109.0 for those with asthma. After taking age, sex, ethnic origin, comorbid conditions, and the use of immunotherapeutic treatments into account, the risk of undergoing an anaphylactic reaction for those with asthma was still elevated 5.2 times (95% confidence interval, 4.7–5.6) above the background risk. Asthmatics also had a statistically elevated risk of developing three other allergic conditions, ranging from 1.4- to 1.9-fold enhanced risk. Severity of asthma is also correlated significantly with the risk of foodstuff-associated, insect venom-associated, and NOS causes of anaphylaxis [277].

A study by Gonzalez-Perez et al. [278] looked at how common anaphylaxis was in patients with asthma, separated into severe or non-severe subgroups. Compared with non-asthmatics, those with asthma overall are at greater risk of anaphylaxis (50.45 as against 21.28 per 100,000 people-years). Similarly, severe asthma conferred greater risk of anaphylaxis than non-severe asthma: 65.35 vs. 43.01 per 100,000 people-years. If we compare the two groups with non-asthmatics, severe asthma increased anaphylactic events by 3.3, non-severe asthma by 2. Being female confers greater risk, most noticeably in the severe asthma group [278].

2.4.3 Allergic Rhinitis and Anaphylaxis

Allergic rhinitis has a prevalence of approximately 10–20% and may be continual or periodic. Nasal pruritus, sternutation, blocked nose and nasal discharge comprise the symptoms. It may co-occur with allergic conjunctivitis (ophthalmic pruritus and lacrimation are the usual symptoms). Mast cells degranulate, triggering an inflammatory cascade that may result in oedema sufficient to obstruct the ostia of the sinuses and Eustachian tubes, putting the patient at risk of an opportunistic bacterial infection. Within the nose, polyps may form, which are composed of mucosa wrapped around an inflammatory exudate. Avoiding the allergenic trigger may prove troublesome; hence, the mainstay of therapy lies in daily use of H1-specific antihistamines which are non-sedating (terfenadine, loratidine, and cetirizine are three such), together with topical steroid ointments (beclometasone) for allergic rhinitis and sodium cromoglycate eyedrops for allergic conjunctivitis. Whilst desensitising treatments are unusual, where a single antigen accounts for the symptoms, or the condition is refractory, desensitisation may have a role to play. Peptide analogues for the epitopes responsible are under evaluation as a means of immunisation. Their mechanism of action involves modulating the Th2-modulated allergic cascade. Cat fur and house dust mite have known epitopes, and these are being evaluated, but clinical use so far is limited [266].

2.4.3.1 Pathophysiology

The nasal, conjunctival, Eustachian, middle ear, sinusal, and pharyngeal mucosae are all subject to an inflammatory response in allergic rhinitis. Nasal involvement is invariable, but the other surfaces are variable affected. The resulting inflammatory responses are characterised by complexity of intercellular signalling, but share the common trigger of IgE complexing with an extrinsic protein to initiate the cascade [279, 280].

An allergic diathesis (i.e. the propensity to react to extrinsic allergenic substances through the formation of IgE) is partly genetically based. Individuals who have this tendency become sensitised to extrinsic proteins, a response caused by IgE to that allergen being expressed. IgE is spread over the surface membrane of mastocytes located within the mucosa of the nasal lining. Inhaled allergen (e.g. pollen of a particular species) is bound by mast cell IgE, resulting in acute degranulation and further mediators being released after a delay [280–282]. Histamine, tryptase, chymase, kinins, and heparin are involved in the initial degranulation [281, 282]. Mastocytes then rapidly switch to the production of other signal molecules such as the leukotrienes and prostaglandin D2 [283–285]. It is the latter which account for the symptoms associated with nasal discharge (blockage, sternutation, pruritus, erythema, nasal tears, oedema, otic pressure, and postnasal drip), through their actions on the cascade. Mucous glands receive a stimulus to increase secretory activity. Vascular endothelium becomes more permeable, with an exudate forming. The vasodilated vessels contribute to nasal blockage and increased pressures. Sternutation and pruritus are mediated through excitation of sensory nerves. Such responses happen within minutes of allergenic contact, being termed the early (immediate) reaction phase [279].

Within the next 4–8 h, mediator release triggers a complex orchestrated response involving multiple inflammatory cellular agents approaching the mucosa: neutrophils, eosinophils, lymphocytes, and macrophages [286]. Thus the inflammatory response persists (late reaction phase). There is some symptomatic overlap between phases, but the late reaction triggers nasal blockage and mucus discharge to a greater extent than sternutation and pruritus, the reverse pattern of the early reaction [286]. Late phase duration is from hours to days, with generalised symptoms (debility, somnolence, and malaise) attributable to the immune system's actions. These systemic symptoms are frequent causes of a decreased quality of life [279].

2.4.3.2 Symptoms and Chronicity

The age at which symptoms first appeared should be noted, together with an indication of how persistent they are. The majority of sufferers from allergic rhinitis have their first episode by the age of 20, although some first episodes happen only long after adolescence [287].

The chronological course of the illness should also be noted, with particular reference to persistence (implying perennial variant) or intermittent (implying seasonal variant of rhinitis), or features implying both types. For flare-ups, it is worth establishing whether the patient has the symptoms every day, or merely on occasion. Within a day, do symptoms remain present all the time or at certain times? Recording such details informs the diagnosis and helps identify the allergen [279].

Note down the pattern of organ involvement and the details of symptoms. A subgroup of hay fever sufferers have symptoms confined nasally, whilst the other subgroup's symptoms involve various organs.

Certain cases of rhinitis—the archetypal ones—exhibit sternutation, pruritus, excessive lacrimation, and watery nasal discharge, but more atypical presentations may consist of nasal blockage alone. If nasal blockage is very marked and confined to one nostril, suspicions should be aroused that there is an actual structural obstruction, e.g. bent septum, polyp, or foreign object [279].

2.4.3.3 Trigger Factors

It is important to decide on the chronological relationship between triggers and symptoms. Examples could be pollen inhalation outside the home, fungal spore exposure when working in gardens, coming into contact with particular animals or house dust raised during cleaning. Exposure to irritant substances from smoking, polluted air, or powerful odours may exacerbate pre-existing hay fever symptoms as well as being a common cause for nasal discharge in themselves. Hay fever with irritant-induced nasal discharge is a common combination. Perennial symptoms in the absence of a recognisable trigger are sometimes described, which may represent a rhinitis of a cause other than allergy, but caution needs to be taken in view of the year-round persistence of some common allergenic sources, such as house dust mites and presence of animals. If symptoms have persisted without a break for a long period, the link with the trigger may have been obscured [279].

Taking a detailed account from the patient that covers all possible environmental allergens, the patients may encounter (not excluding year-round exposure to e.g. fungal spores, house dust mites, and animals) will assist in identifying the source of allergen [288, 289]. House dust mite exposure is more common in homes with carpets, extra warmth, humid atmospheres, and bedding lacking protective covers. Houses that are continually damp increase the risk of exposure to mould. Leaning about a patient's hobbies and leisure pursuits permits evaluation of pollen exposure risks and probable time course. History needs to focus on the domestic and occupational environment with a view to identifying more general year-round triggers such as mites, mould or pets alongside occupation-linked triggers such as laboratory animals, products made from animals, grains and organic substances like wood dust, rubber, and enzymes [279].

2.4.3.4   Comorbid Conditions

Sufferers from hay fever may also have further allergic disorders such as asthma [290, 291] or eczema [292]. Some 20% of hay fever sufferers are also asthmatic. If hay fever is inadequately controlled, asthma may deteriorate [293], as may eczema [292]. This fact should be borne in mind when taking down the patient's account [279].

It is important to check for hay fever complications, a frequent example of which is sinusitis. Potential complications include middle ear infections, sleep problems, apnoea, dental complications (overbite), and abnormality of the palate [294]. The presence of any complications may force an alteration in treatment plan. Nasal polyposis is found to occur with hay fever, but the degree to which this association represents causality is moot. Medical treatments may be insufficient to resolve polyp formation and may increase the risk of sinusitis or sleep disturbance for patients [279].

Take careful note of previous medical problems, not forgetting ongoing medical issues. Rhinitis of the non-allergic type may be secondary to some other conditions, e.g. hypothyroidism or sarcoidosis. Comorbidity can affect treatment choices in prescribing. One case–control study based on a population of children uncovered a powerful association between allergic problems and ADHD (attention-deficit/hyperactivity disorder). There were 4692 cases of ADHD and 18,768 control cases, obtained through randomisation. The ADHD children were more prone to allergic problems in general, particularly hay fever and allergic conjunctivitis [279, 295].

2.4.3.5 Mortality/Morbidity

Allergic rhinitis does not by itself have an associated mortality except if severe asthma or anaphylaxis co-occurs. However, it does have a fair degree of associated morbidity. The coexistence of hay fever and asthma is frequent in patients and hay fever may cause asthmatic flare-ups [290, 291, 293].

There are associations between hay fever and middle ear infections, abnormal functioning of the Eustachian tubes, sinusitis, nasal polyposis, allergic conjunctivitis, and allergic eczema [266, 279, 292]. These conditions add to the burden of morbidity and may even lead to death [279]. There is a synergy between uncontrolled inflammation in hay fever and inflammatory processes occurring in asthma [290, 291, 293] and eczema [292], which may explain the increased morbidity and greater risk of dying [279]. More generally, hay fever may worsen sleep problems, exacerbate learning disabilities and cause fatigue [296–298].

Hay fever not infrequently decreases patients' quality of life. The symptoms of debility and somnolence produced either by the disorder or its treatment can damage performance in study or occupationally lead to absences from school or work and may cause traffic accidents. A recent estimate of the entire economic costs (directly or indirectly caused) attributable to allergic rhinitis gave an annual figure of $5.3 billion [279, 299].

2.5   Anaphylaxis Related to Intravenous Drug Administration

2.5.1   Background

Allergic reactions to drugs fall under type B reactions of the adaptive immune system. Clinically distinguishing between allergic and other types of drug reaction is frequently complex. Given that the signs and symptoms of an allergic drug reaction are only visible when a response is occurring and not when the initial sensitisation takes place, the scientific consensus has been that allergic drug reactions can only happen if the patient is re-exposed to a drug or if administration has lasted a minimum period of 3 days. Newer data have shown, nonetheless, that previous exposure to the causative agent is not a necessary condition for hypersensitivity of the immune system to that agent [300–303]. Such data necessitate a change in scientific reasoning, and it is now evident that a better explanation may be that an allergy to a different xenobiotic acquired earlier causes a cross-reaction in the patient [300].

2.5.2   Sensitisation to Drugs

2.5.2.1   T-Cell Sensitisation

The small size of drugs prevents them acting alone as immunogens, and therefore, they must instead be haptens or prohaptens, chemically active compounds of low molecular weight (typically under 1000 daltons) which are complex to higher molecular weight proteins or peptides to produce an immune response. Haptens do this directly, but prohaptens are first metabolised into an active form that is then capable of covalent bonding with the larger carrier molecule, a process termed bioactivation [304, 305]. Hapten-carrier molecules (complexed drug and protein/peptide) are absorbed by cells capable of presenting antigen (APCs), which then home to the lymphatic drainage system and, after processing the hapten-carrier, display it on MHC (major histocompatibility) membrane proteins, at which point T-cell sensitisation can happen. Non-committed T-cells which have a corresponding specificity recognise the MHC-hapten-carrier complex and undergo reproductive division, to become primed T-cells [306]. From this lineage spring short-lived T-cells of the effector subtype (T_{eff}) alongside the long-lived T-cell subtypes: effector memory (T_{EM}) and central memory (T_{CM}). Each subpopulation has a predilection for a specific tissue: uncommitted and T_{CM} populations home to lymph nodes, whilst effector populations (T_{Eff} and T_{EM}) have the ability to go to tissues expressing particular ligands [308]. These latter presumably home to where the hapten-carrier complex was first found [300].

2.5.2.2   Antibody Sensitisation

Hapten-carrier compounds may be able to stimulate both T- and B-cells. If committed T-cells are available to assist, B-cells with specificity for a drug may undergo division and differentiation into plasmocytes, which then express immunoglobulins of various types versus the drug. If Th2 cells (T-helper subtype 2) are present, which express IL4, IL5, and IL10, IgE is the favoured isotype. If cytokines produced by Th1 predominate, IgG and IgM expression wins out [300].

2.5.2.3   Cross-Reactivity

Alongside hapten and prohapten carrier compounds formed with drugs, there can be haptens and pro-haptens unrelated to drugs that cause a hypersensitivity to drugs by cross-reactivity of allergens. That such a mechanism must exist has been evidenced by new research. About 17 patients out of a cohort of 25 (i.e. 68%) who had had anaphylaxis to cetuximab actually already had serum antibodies to the drug before any treatment had commenced. The immunoglobulins in question had an affinity for galactose-α-1,3-galactose, located on the fragment antigen-binding section of the heavy chain of the cetuximab molecule [301]. This antigen shares multiple similarities with molecules forming part of the ABO blood grouping system. In addition, exposure to pholcodine led to the development of IgE specific to morphine, as well as suxamethonium, an agent involved in cases of allergy to neuromuscular blockers [302]. In cases where patients had both clinically confirmed drug allergy and skin-testing positivity to contrast media containing iodine, half of such cases had reacted on first exposure to the medium yet had never come across it before [303]. There are also accounts in the literature of food or cosmetic products having occasioned a cross-reaction with a specific drug [300, 309].

2.5.3 Immune-Mediated Drug Sensitivity

2.5.3.1 IgE-Mediated Drug Hypersensitivity (Type I)

If a drug when first given has produced sensitivity and IgE production, even low volumes of the antigenic drug may trigger allergic symptoms. The reason for such highly tuned sensitivity to antigen is the very widespread distribution in the body of mast cells expressing Fc (fragment, crystallisable) receptors (FcεRI), which bind IgE to the antigen with great affinity. It is currently held necessary for antigen to be in an aggregated form to elicit the reaction. In allergy, the Fab (fragment antigen-binding) section of immunoglobulin E is bound to the epitope, and when at least two IgE molecules have bound to the allergen, cross-linking can take place, causing mast cells to degranulate their contents of histamine, and secrete the leukotrienes, prostaglandins, and cytokines. This secretion of signalling molecules leads to dilatation of blood vessels, enhanced permeability of endothelium, increased mucus production, constriction of the airways, as well as drawing eosinophils into the affected regions. Whilst allergic drug reactions frequently cause hives or angioedema, symptoms affecting breathing, producing shock and extreme compromise to the heart are also possible. Type I reactions often result from penicillins, cephalosporins, and neuromuscular blockers [300].

2.5.3.2   IgG-Mediated Cytotoxicity (Type II)

Type II reactions are characterised by IgG involvement, which causes injury to red blood cells, white cells, thrombocytes, and, it is likely, precursor cells in bone marrow responsible for haematopoiesis. Some typical culprits are methyldopa, which results in haemolytic anaemia; aminopyrine that caused leucocytopaenia; and heparin which may deplete platelets. Cells targeted are coated by IgG and then the liver and spleen (reticuloendothelial) system sequesters the targets by binding via Fc or the complement receptor. Less often, cytolysis may occur within the blood vessels as a result of the action of the complement cascade.

There have been several proposed explanations of how T-cells recognise their target antibody [310, 311]. Two pathways are put forward: in the first, alterations to membrane structure due to drug (hapten) generate the immune response against the target; in the second, haptens cause cell membranes to undergo a change in conformation, and this then allows non-specific autoantibodies (not specific to the hapten) to target the cell as a whole. This second pathway should then only be active whilst soluble hapten persists [300].

2.5.3.3   Immune Complex Deposition (Type III)

It is frequent for immune complexes to be formed in adaptive immune responses, and symptoms are not generally caused thereby. Somewhat rarely, these immune complexes may bind to endothelium, causing complexes to be deposited within small diameter vessels and the complement cascade to be triggered. The reasons for this and the precipitating factors remain unknown. Clinically, type III reactions present as serum sickness, lupus erythematosus, or vasculitis, for example agents triggering these events being, respectively, β-lactams, quinidine and minocycline [300].

2.5.3.4   T-Cell-Mediated Drug Hypersensitivity (Type IV)

T-cell-mediated drug hypersensitivity can result in several different clinical pictures, at one end of the spectrum, skin involvement alone, at the other severe generalised disease. Sulpha antimicrobials and β-lactams are often implicated [300].

2.5.4   Drug-Induced Anaphylactic Reactions

Anaphylaxis, which can cause death, is a rare type of hypersensitivity reaction. European incidence is between 1.5 and 7.9 per 100,000 person-years [312]. Data on hospital admissions suggest an incidence of 1.95 per 100,000 person-years [313]. After adjustment for age, the incidence in the US is 6.6 for males and 8.7 for females, each per 100,000 person-years [314]. Anaphylaxis has an abrupt onset following allergenic exposure [315]. It is hard to distinguish anaphylactic from anaphylactoid reactions on clinical observations alone. An anaphylactoid reaction occurs without prior sensitisation and is non-immune in origin. Mast cells and basophils degranulate in response to non-immune triggers. The treatment of both anaphylactic and anaphylactoid reactions does not differ.

Substances that frequently trigger anaphylaxis are medications, foodstuffs, bites and stings by insects, radiological contrast agents, and latex rubber [315, 317]. Amongst medications, antibiotics, NSAIDs, and muscle relaxants are frequently the agents responsible [317, 318]. Currently there are no tests or risk stratification procedures capable of sorting out cases at risk of anaphylaxis from those at risk of less severe allergic responses. One exception in this regard is asthmatics, whose allergic reactions tend to be more severe [316].

According to Patel et al. [319], reporting from Indian data, as previous international studies have shown [318, 320–322], antibiotics are the most frequent medications causing anaphylaxis. Of the antibiotics, β-lactams are of especial concern [317, 318, 320–324]. In a multi-national collaborative study, they caused anaphylaxis in between 5.7 and 32 of the 100,000 individuals exposed to them [325]. Within the beta-lactam class itself, amoxicillin [318, 320, 321] and co-amoxyclav [326] as well as the cephalosporins [322] were most frequently cited. A study performed in Italy reported on the odds ratio for anaphylaxis with several antimicrobials in frequent use: penicillins 1.64 (1.30–2.05), cephalosporins 2.36 (1.76–3.17), glycopeptides 2.46 (1.14–5.30), and quinolones 2.17 (1.69–2.79) [317]. In calculating odds ratios, a case definition of anaphylaxis with the drug suspected was used, with controls as the number of non-anaphylactic drug reactions for the same agent. The Indian study identified artesunate as the second most frequent antimicrobial implicated. This conflicts with the data reported from Europe [317, 318, 321–323], but may be due to its high frequency of use in India as an anti-malarial. That IgE plays a role in artesunate allergy was confirmed by skin testing [319].

In the scientific literature, diclofenac is the most common allergen amongst NSAIDs [321]. Diclofenac was the only NSAID in the Italian study to have an odds ratio that reached statistical significance at 3.23 (95% CI: 2.21–4.73) [317]. Van Puijenbroek et al. estimated the odds ratio for diclofenac to cause an anaphylactic reaction as 17.2 (95% CI: 12.1–24.5), a ratio appreciably above that of other NSAIDs [327]. Looking at diclofenac and comparing various routes of administration gives incidence ratios of oral, 7.2 (2.6–20), parenteral, 9.0 (2.7–30), and suppository, 16 (3.4–74) per 100,000 exposed patients, in each case the numbers in parentheses specifying the 95% confidence interval [325]. Amongst NSAIDs, we can distinguish between two groups with variable odds ratios, distinguished by their chemical makeup: heteroaryl acids (diclofenac, tolmetin, and ketorolac) had a collective odds ratio of 19.7 (95% CI: 13.8–28.1), higher than the arylpropionic acid group (ibuprofen, naproxen, flurbiprofen, ketoprofen, fenoprofen, and oxaprozin) with OR of 6.7 (95% CI: 4.2–10.6). By contrast, Renaudin et al. [318] identified paracetamol and ibuprofen as higher risk agents, and Moro et al. picked out ibuprofen and acetylsalicylic acid as their highest risk agents.

Neuromuscular blockade with rocuronium, succinylcholine, atracurium, and vecuronium is associated frequently with anaphylaxis in reports [118, 318, 323, 328, 329]. A study focusing on anaphylaxis that resulted in death in the UK revealed that drug-related anaphylaxis exerted its effect through the cardiovascular system, whilst foodstuff-related anaphylaxis exerted its effects through the respiratory system [252].

2.5.5   Clinical Manifestations

Genuine allergy-related drug responses mimic other diseases significantly and can affect every organ system, or be generalised, as with anaphylaxis. A common presentation of drug reaction is as a skin alteration, as the skin plays an important role in immune and metabolic processes, the most common of all being morbilliform eruptions. A red, maculopapular exanthem confined initially to the trunk, may appear around 1–3 weeks following commencing a medication, and then spreads to arms and legs. Hives are generally a sign of a true allergy of type I, but are possible in a type III reaction or in pseudoallergy. Extreme drug sensitivity reactions that are non-allergenic and affect the skin (i.e., erythema multiforme, Stevens–Johnson syndrome, and toxic epidermal necrolysis) are blistering skin pathologies necessitating urgent diagnosis and treatment due to heavy morbidity and threat to life. Contact dermatitis is principally in response to local applications of drug and resembles eczema. It is a type IV reaction [330].

Drug hypersensitivity needs to be considered as a diagnosis in cases even where the typical allergic symptomatology (anaphylaxis, hives, and asthma) is not present. Such cases may present with symptoms resembling serum sickness, exanthemata, pyrexia, pulmonary infiltrates, raised eosinophil blood count, hepatitis, acute interstitial nephritis, and symptoms that resemble SLE. Diagnosing drug hypersensitivity entails a search for symptoms and signs consistent with the diagnosis [330].

Because of their shared molecular structure involving the β-lactam ring and ensuing cross-reactivity, an allergy to penicillin is a relative contraindication to the use of carbapenems [331]. (The evidence supporting this conclusion is a non-randomised trial, therefore level B.) However, aztreonam (Azactam) rarely causes cross-reactivity in penicillin-allergic patients [332, 333]. The cross-reactions between cephalosporins and penicillins have been reported at various levels. From 1980 onwards, reports have indicated that cross-reactions between penicillin and second- or third-generation cephalosporins occur with at most 5% frequency [334]. First-generation cephalosporins seemingly have a greater propensity for cross-reaction [335]. Whilst the actual frequency of cross-reaction between cephalosporins and penicillins is thus low, given that allergic response may result in life-threatening anaphylaxis [154], a cautious approach to prescribing cephalosporins to penicillin-allergic patients is to be recommended. One way to mitigate the risk is to perform cutaneous testing for penicillin first, especially if a previous allergic reaction has been extreme [336, 337].

The older cephalosporins (first generation: cephalothin, cephalexin, cefadroxil) possess a molecular geometry more similar to penicillin than newer agents (cefprozil, cefuroxime, ceftazidime, ceftriaxone) which lack the antigenic side chain and for this reason the older agents have a greater propensity to cause an allergic cross-reaction [338].

One report has questioned the 10% figure for anaphylactic cross-reactivity cited in much of the literature, substituting a tentative 1%, and observing that most such reactions were classifiable as mild [339]. A study based on review of hospital admission records related to patients with a documented penicillin allergy who subsequently went on to receive a cephalosporin noted that out of 606 such cases, only a single case resulted in allergic response (i.e. 0.17%), which was also minor [340].

A different study, though, paints a different picture: being allergic to penicillin confers an approximately threefold enhanced risk of allergic response to drugs in general, whilst the risk of reacting against cephalosporins in patients known to be allergic to penicillin is approaching eight times that of patients with no such allergy. One explanation for this is that, rather than a true cross-reactivity, what is being observed is a general hyper-responsivity by the immune system, at least to some extent [335].

If a patient whose condition mandates emergency treatment to avoid loss of life would ideally receive either a penicillin or cephalosporin, several courses of action are possible. If the account of an allergy is not certain, a closely monitored trial of the drug may be attempted, although whenever possible, clinicians should involve the patient and obtain consent. Anaphylactic resuscitation facilities should be at hand. If the account is more definite, choice of a different medication must be undertaken, provided it has a comparable efficacy. Failing both these, desensitisation is the only option [338].

There are multiple agents other than antibiotics with a propensity to induce anaphylaxis through the formation of specific IgE, but anaphylaxis with these agents is less frequent. Within surgical departments, anaphylaxis is typically attributable to muscle relaxants; however, the possibility of a reaction to hypnotics, antibiotics, opioids, colloids, and other agents needs to be considered. During the 1980s there was a surge in latex allergy reports in response to the adoption of universal precautions (using latex gloves, etc.) in an era of HIV, Hep B and C epidemics, but new cases are now less frequent following the wider use of non-latex materials. Where latex does provoke anaphylaxis perioperatively, the anaphylaxis generally occurs whilst anaesthesia is being maintained rather than at induction. Induction-related anaphylaxis is usually due to substances other than latex. Whilst inhaled agents of anaesthesia can be toxic to the liver through an immune reaction, they have not been linked to anaphylaxis thus far [341].

2.5.5.1 Immunological Reactions to Aspirin, NSAIDs, and ACE Inhibitors

Traditionally, reactions to aspirin and the NSAIDs (non-steroidal anti-inflammatory drugs) have been considered not to be mediated through IgE, but instead to represent a perturbation of arachidonic acid metabolism [338]. Skin eruptions in isolation following aspirin or NSAIDs, together with spasm of the bronchi (frequently with polyp formation in the nose) in the subgroup of asthma sufferers with sensitivity to aspirin is, however, mediated through IgE. The inhibition of cyclooxygenase by this group of agents blocks the prostanoid pathway and results in overexpression of leukotrienes by the activity of the 5-lipoxygenase pathway. Such individuals show a high degree of cross-reactions between aspirin and most of the NSAID agents [338].

The occurrence of anaphylaxis following NSAID or aspirin administration is, nonetheless, due to a pathophysiological process that involves IgE. In genuine anaphylaxis, there is no apparent cross-reaction between the different agents that all block cyclooxygenase. Moreover, anaphylaxis depends on a minimum of double exposure to the drug, a feature consistent with the sensitisation hypothesis. As a last consideration, patients whose reaction is unequivocally anaphylactic seldom have comorbid asthma, nasal polyp formation, or hives [338].

ACEi agents (angiotensin-converting enzyme inhibitors), which are frequently employed to manage hypertension, cause between 0.5 and 1 in 100 patients to develop angioedema. But anaphylaxis is a rare response to these medications [338].

2.5.5.2 Immunological IgE-Independent Reactions

Blood products (e.g. intravenous immunoglobulin, animal-derived antiserum) can produce anaphylaxis, due in part to complement activation. The complement cascade can then trigger mast cell and basophils to degranulate [338].

2.5.5.3   Exercise-Induced Anaphylaxis

Anaphylaxis brought on by exercise is seldom encountered, but occurs in two variants. In the first of these, certain foodstuffs (e.g. wheat or celery) or medications (e.g. NSIDs) must have been ingested shortly before exercising for the syndrome to be initiated. In such cases, the ingestion of the substance or the exercise can be enjoyed separately without inducing anaphylaxis. In the second type, anaphylaxis can occur from time to time when exercising and is not linked to food being eaten. Exercise is not an invariable trigger for anaphylaxis in these patients. These kinds of anaphylaxis may be a symptom of mastocytosis, in which mast cell numbers are abnormally elevated in several organs. Allergic reactions to food or insect venoms are more likely in individuals with mastocytosis. It is usual to advise the patient to avoid substances that can potentially cause the degranulation of mast cells on their own, such as alcohol, vancomycin, opiate medications, radiological contrast media, and certain other biologics [338].

2.5.5.4   Non-immunological Reactions

It is believed that some drugs (amongst which are opioids, dextrans, protamine, and vancomycin) can induce mediator release from mast cells without any immune system mediation. There is also some evidence to support the hypothesis that dextrans and protamine have the ability to initiate the action of certain pathways for inflammation, such as the complement cascade, clotting pathway, and the kallikrein–kinin (vasoactive) system [338].

Radio-contrastive agents given intravenously may provoke an anaphylactoid reaction which resembles genuine anaphylaxis clinically and indeed is managed identically. There is no relationship with previous exposure to the medium. Around 1–3 in a hundred patients who are administered hyperosmolar IV contrast develop reactions, but most reactions are mild (typically urticaria occurs) and seldom threaten life. The associated mortality from IV contrast usage is calculated to be 0.9 cases per 100,000 instances of use [338].

Prophylactic administration of antihistamines or steroids coupled with lower molecular weight (LMW) agents has reduced the level of anaphylactoid reactions in contrast procedures to around 0.5%. Given that the rate of reaction following a first reaction is estimated to leap up to 17–60%, it is worth contemplating the use of prophylaxis in patients with a previous reaction. The use of LMW agents alone prevails in some units. Appropriate staff members, drugs, and equipment in case of an allergic reaction should be assembled prior to contrast administration, and the patient's agreement obtained in advance of the procedure [338].

Patients with an allergic diathesis or asthma have a greater chance of reacting. Beta-blockade makes allergy more likely to be treatment resistant. But allergies to shellfish or iodine do not necessarily mean prophylaxis must be administered. As is the case with all allergy sufferers, LMW contrast agent usage should be considered. An allergy to iodine alone is not in fact possible, since iodine is essential in trace quantities for life. The term is misleading, with most patients who report such allergies found on careful consideration to have experienced contrast reactions, shellfish allergy, or contact injury from povidone-iodine (Betadine). Since exposure of the patient to contrast medium solely across a mucous membrane has not yet resulted in anaphylactic reactions, the genitourinary or gastrointestinal use of radio-contrast agents is still permissible where previous reaction via parenteral administration has occurred [338].

2.5.6   *Laboratory Evaluation*

Laboratory tests aim to measure biochemical and immunological parameters which can confirm or disconfirm that a specific immune pathway lies behind a suspected adverse drug event. The putative mechanism should guide the tests undertaken [330, 342].

To confirm a reaction due to type I hypersensitivity, IgE to specific antigen is measured. Cutaneous testing is of use in this diagnosis. There are standard clinical testing protocols for suspected penicillin allergy as well as well-established procedures for testing local anaesthetic [343] and muscle relaxant [344] hypersensitivities. Skin testing also helps with the identification of larger molecular antigens such as insulin, some vaccines, streptokinase, antibodies (poly- or monoclonal), and latex rubber [345, 346]. If the test is positive, it confirms that specific IgE is being produced and is consistent with a clinical diagnosis of type I hypersensitivity. If the test is negative, this currently only confirms that penicillin allergy is not present, since others lack adequate sensitivity so far [347]. A negative cutaneous testing result cannot exclude that IgE specific to that drug does in fact occur. For a restricted range of drugs, an alternative radioallergosorbent (RAST) test is available, although now its sensitivity has been up to below that of cutaneous tests. Since the epitopes of many medications are not known, this limits the tests' ability to predict clinical response [348].

If taken less than 4 h after the allergic response, mast cell activation levels measured in vitro are of value. Histamine levels in the blood are at a maximum 5 min post anaphylactic reaction, but go back to normal in under half an hour. Tryptase in the blood is at a maximum 1 h post event, staying high for between 2 and 4 h [349]. Whilst histamine, tryptase, and betatryptase measurement have been of use to verify an acute allergic response occurring through IgE, normal levels may still be measured even in genuine allergic responses [334, 350]. The haemolytic anaemia, thrombocytopenia, or neutropenia associated with type II reactions should result in an abnormal full blood count. Coombs' direct or indirect test can verify a haemolytic anaemia if positive. This test checks for complement activity (with or without hapten) binding to erythrocytes [330].

Type III reactions (which involve formation of immune complexes) to medications may be associated with rises in the general markers of inflammation, such as erythrocyte sedimentation and C-reactive protein. Where facilities for testing exist, complement proteins can be measured directly (CH50, C3, C4), as can the level of immune complexes in the blood. Positive testing has a value in confirmation of a clinical diagnosis, but negativity does not permit the exclusion of a type III reaction. The occurrence of generalised vasculitis secondary to drugs can be verified by antinuclear or antihistone antibody titres [351].

Type IV reactions classically occur in the form of allergic eczematous eruptions secondary to topical application. The area may be indurated and reddened, with a vesiculopapular exanthem that causes itching and appears 48 h after a patch has been applied. Such features lend weight to a diagnosis of type IV reaction [330].

2.5.7   Treatment

The single most important step to manage and treat a drug hypersensitivity is to stop the drug responsible, wherever practicable. If a suitable substitute drug exists that has a different chemical structure, it can be used as a replacement. However, close monitoring of the clinical effects of stopping and swapping will be needed. For most cases, assuming the diagnosis of hypersensitivity is right, the symptoms will abate within a fortnight [352].

Other forms of treatment for such reactions are, for the most part, palliative in intention. If the reaction is extreme, systemic steroid administration may quicken the resolution of symptoms. Steroidal creams and histamine blockers given orally can help with cutaneous symptom resolution. Stevens–Johnson syndrome and toxic epidermal necrolysis, which are of grave severity, necessitate further clinically intense measures [352].

The chapter dealing with anaphylaxis provides further details on the treatment of anaphylactic reactions.

2.6   Exercise-Induced Anaphylaxis

2.6.1   *Background*

Exercise-induced anaphylaxis (EIA) describes a clinical syndrome in which anaphylaxis is brought on by physical exertion [353]. Itching, urticaria, flushed skin, wheezing, and gastrointestinal symptoms such as nausea, griping, and diarrhoea are symptomatic of this condition. If the triggering activity does not stop, the symptoms may worsen in severity, with angioedema, swelling of the larynx, a fall in blood pressure, and finally, cardiovascular collapse. On the other hand, stopping the activity in question generally leads to instant amelioration of the symptomatology [354].

Sheffer and Austen identified, in their series of 16 patients, all of whom had EIA and whose ages ranged from 12 to 54, four distinct phases, which they labelled "prodromal", "early", "fully established", and "late" [355]. The prodrome was characterised by the patients feeling fatigued, sensing they were warm and itching all over, and reddening of the skin. The early phase had a characteristic systemic hives response. Once fully established, patients described choking, noisy breath sounds, abdominal griping pains, the desire to vomit, and actual vomiting. Late symptoms could last for between 1 and 3 days after and might, for example, comprise a headache over the temples [354].

Exercise of greater intensity (jogging, playing tennis, dance moves, cycling) is more usual preceding an attack than less intense activity such as going for a walk or gardening, but both may precede symptoms. A study with a lengthy tracking period identified jogging as the most frequent antecedent for EIA [356]. A selection of reports have identified running, playing football, collecting leaves, moving piles of snow, and horse riding as triggers [357].

For food-related EIA, wheat, shellfish, tomatoes, groundnuts, and corn are the most frequent accompaniments [358], but other foods have also been implicated, such as fruit, seeds, milk, soya, lettuce, peas, beans, rice, and meat of different types [353].

Allergens that have been inhaled rather than ingested are also associated with EIA. A case report mentions a male aged 14 who had an episode of extreme EIA following eating food that had *Penicillium* mould growing on it and who then ran at school [358]. A further case report describes a female aged 16 with EIA following eating wheat flour infested with grain mites [359].

Evidence for a genetic form of the disorder comes from families in which several members have had EIA and have an allergic diathesis [360]. A total of seven individuals, all male, from three generations of a family, each had skin and breathing symptoms of allergy induced by exercise [361].

Maulitz et al. [362] wrote a case report on an individual who experienced anaphylaxis twice following running. Both times shellfish had been consumed between 5 and 24 h earlier. Neither shellfish nor heavy exercise alone could replicate the symptoms. Kidd and colleagues [363] offered four similar examples, giving the syndrome the title "Food-dependent, exercise-induced anaphylaxis" (FDEIA).

Sheffer and Austen, in their 1980 paper, wrote about a case series of 16 individuals. These people suffered a number of symptoms of anaphylaxis, such as whole body hives, itching, angioedema, abdominal griping, and low blood pressure following exercising [355]. Given the similarities with anaphylaxis as a result of allergenic exposure, they offered the label "exercise induced anaphylaxis" [364].

Around 5–15% of the total cases of anaphylaxis are instances of EIA, it is thought [365]. Whilst cases of FDEIA are underreported, the prevalence has been put at between 1 in 3 and 1 in 2 of EIA cases. Based on a sample exceeding 76,000 in size of Japanese schoolchildren at junior high school, only 24 cases of EIA (0.031%) and 13 of FDEIA (0.017%) were identified by Aihara et al. [357].

2.6.2 Epidemiology

Precise determinations of the prevalence of EIA and FDEIA are not yet available. Whilst the distribution of disorders is worldwide [356, 357, 366], not many investigations to determine the true prevalence in a systematic way have been undertaken. A study using a questionnaire to poll 76,229 Japanese junior high school children gave a prevalence of EIA as 0.03% and FDEIA as 0.017% [357], whilst an older study, also from Japan, gave a higher figure (0.21%) for FDEIA in a comparable population [366]. EIA and FDEIA are generally isolated cases; however, a familial type has also been identified [360, 361]. There was a 2:1 female:male predilection in a large cohort of 279 cases of EIA [385], but a different study did not identify such a trend [357].

2.6.3 Pathophysiology

The underlying pathological mechanism behind EIA and FDEIA remains unclear. What role (or roles) exercise plays in triggering the episodes is unknown [367].

Mast cells in the skin are known to degranulate, and circulating levels of histamine [368] and tryptase [369] to rise, in EIA. It has been postulated, therefore, that, just as with other types of anaphylaxis, mast cells would degranulate upon activation in EIA, but the level of stimulus required for degranulation to occur would be lower in EIA. How this lowering occurs, from a cellular or physiological point of view, is not yet evident.

One way in which mast cells have been linked to exercise is the known mechanism by which endorphin release occurs during exercise. Endorphins can stimulate mast cell secretion [370]. What role endorphins may play in EIA, though, is still a matter of speculation.

It is implicit in the definition of FDEIA that neither the food trigger nor exercise alone produces problems in sufferers. Accordingly, it has been proposed that the syndrome involves a short-lived loss of normal immunological tolerance brought about by the synergy of exercise and the problem food [354].

Several mechanisms have been suggested to account for FDEIA. The gut becomes more permeable during exercise, which might provide the opportunity for antigenic proteins to cross through to the gastrointestinal outposts of the immune system [371]. NSAIDs and alcohol can facilitate the development of both EIA and FDEIA through enhancing gut permeability [372].

FDEIA might also be linked to autonomic nervous system irregularities. Some research examined autonomic function in four children with FDEIA and compared it with four control subjects [373]. Exercise resulted in greater parasympathetic nervous activity and lower sympathetic responsivity in the cases than in the controls.

Transglutaminase undergoes activation in subjects during exercise. It can bind gliadin (particularly omega-5 gliadin) derived from wheat and thus form higher molecular weight complexes capable of stimulating an immune response, involving IgE binding and cross-linkage [374]. According to this model, exercise-induced alterations in the processing of allergens may increase their allergenic potential.

It is known, e.g. from studying groundnut allergy, that the ease with which an epitope can be recognised plays a role in modulating how severely allergic a patient becomes [375]. Processes peculiar to exercise may enhance the recognition of allergen by the immune system.

Exercising causes the mobilisation and activation of cells of immune origin within the gut and perturbs the usual balance between pro- and anti-inflammatory responses [376]. If this process becomes dysregulated in a patient with immune sensitivity to certain foods, the process could be of significance for FDEIA.

In addition, exercising may alter the osmolar gradients in mucosae, causing basophilic release of histamine. One case report reported that a hyperosmolar medium, when given to a patient with known FDEIA caused basophilic discharge of histamine at a greater level than in normal subjects [377].

2.6.4   History

EIA is a syndrome in which signs and symptoms of anaphylaxis occur whilst the patient is engaged in physical exertion. Continuing with the activity worsens the symptoms. Warning signs of an imminent EIA attack are feeling hot all over, itching, reddening of the skin, and diaphoresis. There then develop both urticaria of the usual type and angioedema. The symptoms may develop into gut symptoms, swelling of the larynx, and circulatory collapse [354].

These symptoms may occur at any point during exertion. Stopping the exercise generally leads to the symptoms immediately improving or resolving altogether. A proportion of those affected do, however, continue to progress to circulatory collapse even when the activity has stopped [354].

How often EIA or FDEIA happens when exercising is variable amongst sufferers. Whilst most sufferers exercise on a regular basis, attacks are infrequent. For FDEIA cases, it is characteristic for an attack to happen 1–3 h after eating when engaged in exertion. From beginning exercising to the onset of symptoms can vary between less than 30 min to up to three quarters of an hour [354].

The most frequent signs and symptoms, together with how common they are, are thus [353]:

- Itching (92%)
- Hives (86%)
- Angioedema (72%)
- Becoming red-faced or red elsewhere (70%)
- Dyspnoea (51%)
- Difficulty swallowing (34%)
- Sternal weight (33%)
- Loss of consciousness (32%)
- Diaphoresis (32%)
- Headache (28%)
- Gut symptoms such as feeling need to vomit, diarrhoea, griping (28%)
- Choking, laryngeal constriction, dysphonia (25%)

2.6.5   Physical Examination

Physical examination does not usually find a characteristic pattern in EIA or FDEIA cases. There may be present the stigmata of atopy, such as dermatitis, dark rings around the eyes, and congested nasal passages indicating hay fever [354]. The skin should be carefully examined, looking for signs of dermatographic urticaria or urticaria pigmentosa, indicative of cutaneous mastocytosis. In the latter case, there will be oval to round macules, papules, or raised areas of a reddish-brown colour. Since a possible presentation of mastocytosis is as anaphylaxis brought on by exercise, or by a number of other triggers, being able to remove this from a differential diagnosis is vital [354]. Cardiac auscultation can also exclude exercise-related cardiac dysfunction from the differential diagnosis, if the heart sounds are normal [354].

2.6.6   Diagnosis

EIA is a clinical diagnosis based on history and examination. The diagnosis is made where symptoms of anaphylaxis occur in conjunction with exercise: urticaria, +/− angioedema, or circulatory collapse, in the presence or absence of other symptoms of anaphylaxis, such as gut problems or breathing difficulties affecting any part of the respiratory tree. Having demonstrated the relationship between anaphylaxis and exertion, documentation should unambiguously distinguish between a diagnosis of EIA and FDEIA, since future prevention of such episodes hinges on the diagnosis. Taking a precise history allows EIA to be distinguished from similar-looking episodes of exercise-accompanied anaphylaxis, in which it is not the exercise itself that triggers the anaphylaxis, but some other factor related to the activity, such as cold conditions whilst swimming, taking NSAIDs for analgesia by athletes with energetic schedules, or being in contact with an allergen that itself acts as the trigger (such as latex). Where the history lacks full clarity, consider other possible explanations, since, as clinicians should be aware, a number of other conditions look very similar to anaphylaxis [364].

In children, the differential diagnosis for EIA encompasses cholinergic urticaria, idiopathic cold urticaria, mastocytosis, diseases of the circulatory system, allergy to foodstuffs worsened by exercise, and angioedema [354].

2.6.6.1   Cholinergic Urticaria

Cholinergic urticaria is a type of exogenously triggered urticaria and can be set off through exercising and has characteristic 2–4 mm diameter itching wheals with a surrounding large area of non-raised redness. Occasional case reports describe cases where repeated hypotensive events have resembled EIA [354].

The principal way to tell the disorders apart is the appearance of the skin: cholinergic urticarial hives are very small and may coalesce to form larger hives, whereas EIA hives are extremely large [354]. In addition, the pathological mechanism helps to differentiate the two. Thus, passive heating of the patient leads to different results between the two disorders: in cholinergic urticaria, if the core body temperature rises by greater than seven tenths of a degree (such as in a bath or sauna), histamine release provokes urticaria and symptoms of anaphylaxis; in EIA passive heat fails to trigger an allergic response [354].

2.6.6.2   Idiopathic Cold Urticaria

Idiopathic cold urticaria is a further exogenously triggered urticarial condition in which cold can provoke both hives and angioedema. The disorder may spread to other organs and even to full-blown anaphylaxis. This anaphylactic development has produced mortality directly and indirectly, when cold water swimming ended in drowning [378].

Idiopathic cold urticaria may be wrongly labelled as EIA in patients who complain of symptoms after exerting themselves in a cold environment, if due attention is not paid to whether cold alone is capable of producing symptoms [354].

An ice cube may help to make the diagnosis clearer, since applying one to the skin for a nonspecific period and then allowing the skin to warm back up produces a wheal at the site in idiopathic cold urticaria, but now in EIA [354].

2.6.6.3 Mastocytosis

In mastocytosis, mast cells multiply and increase their levels in a number of organs, most frequently within the skin [379]. Affected patients are at higher risk of anaphylaxis, either from exercising or other causes.

Distinguishing between mastocytosis and EIA/FDEIA can be done biochemically on the basis of blood levels of tryptase. Mastocytosis results in persistently raised levels of serum tryptase, but EIA and FDEIA produce a transient increase only at the time of acute attacks [354]. It can also be done if the patient has oval to round macules, papules, or raised lesions, which are characteristically seen on the skin in urticaria pigmentosa. Unaffected skin when gently stroked develops wheals with pruritic or burning sensations, known as Darier's sign [354].

2.6.6.4 Cardiovascular Disorders

Whilst heart-related events such as heart attack and rhythm disturbances can certainly create fatigue, difficulty breathing, and circulatory collapse whilst a patient is exercising, there would be no accompanying itching, hives, angioedema, or swelling around the larynx [354].

2.6.6.5 Food Allergy Worsened Through Exercise

Exercising may make food allergy reactions worse and happen more often in some patients. The gut wall becomes more permeable during periods of exercise, and this may permit either completely undigested or large fragments of partly digested allergens to enter the blood. To prove that a case is FDEIA rather than food allergy worsened through exercise, formal food challenge can be tried. For the food allergy sufferer this will lead to symptoms, but not for someone with FDEIA [354].

2.6.6.6   Angioedema

Hereditary angioedema is a genetic disorder arising from deficient or non-functioning C1 esterase inhibitor (C1-INH) [380]. The acquired form of the disease is due to pathological autoimmune interaction with C1-INH [381].

Whether hereditary or acquired, angioedema results in repeated angioedema episodes, but no hives or itching, generally affecting the skin or mucosae of the upper respiratory tract and the gut. Physical exertion, stress, or cold weather may trigger an angioedematous episode. The lack of urticaria and itching in both forms of angioedema is a key feature allowing differentiation from EIA [354].

2.6.7   Treatment

Avoiding co-factors: for patients who have a known co-factor that precipitates attacks, the initial step is to avoid the co-factor. For some patients, this approach will be sufficient. Some known co-factors are [382]:

- Non-steroidal anti-inflammatory drugs (NSAIDs)
- Alcohol
- Certain parts of the monthly cycle in women, especially premenstrual or ovulatory phases
- Extreme temperatures (very hot and humid conditions or very cold surroundings)
- Pollens at certain times of year when pollen sensitisation has already occurred

Avoiding food triggers: FDEIA sufferers should not eat the implicated food within 4–6 h of planned physical exertion. An exercise routine that begins before breakfast is a straightforward way to achieve this, albeit one many patients dislike [382].

If the food in question is found in many situations, avoidance may be complicated. A catalogue of foods that are considered "safe" for the patient may be of greater practical use than the admonition to avoid certain foodstuffs and less liable to result in mistaken consumption. Child and adolescent patients especially benefit from such a catalogue. An alternative strategy is for the patients to exclude all consumption of the problem food [369].

For a few cases, even a low-impact form of exercise, such as fast walking may provoke symptoms, preventing proper sequencing of food intake and exertion. In such a situation, dietary exclusion is the only option [382].

Prophylactic prescribing: There is no need to prescribe medication in cases where appropriate behavioural changes and co-factors and problem foods are being avoided. In some cases, however, this may not be achievable and prophylactic prescribing will be needed [382].

Cromoglycates and FDEIA: A number of case reports in the literature posit the use of sodium cromoglycate at high doses by mouth prior to eating as a way to stop attacks happening in cases of FDEIA [383–386]. Such reports involved children and younger adults suffering from FDEIA, who had already been cautioned to avoid exercise for 4 h after food. As an extra measure, for situations in which the patients exercised in the afternoon without prior warning, a dose of sodium cromoglycate was administered 20 min prior to the midday meal [384]. A report on two such children reported success, even where exercise happened unexpectedly after food. Symptoms were confined to periods in which the medication had been forgotten. Both individuals were able to recommence exercise periods after eating, provided they had taken cromoglycate prior to food [384].

Two case reports written about adults with FDEIA related to wheat describe how, in one case, prophylactic cromoglycate stopped wheat allergen being absorbed into the circulation, and in the other case, inhibited the blood histamine level from rising [383]. This report was, nonetheless, contradicted by another one in which, despite administering 100 mg of cromolyn sodium 1 h earlier than food, followed by exercise, doctors were unable to prevent either the development of symptoms or the circulatory absorption of gliadin [387].

H1 blockers: There has been no systematic research into the prophylactic use of H1 blockers to stop EIA. Clinical experience, however, points to its being inconsistent in effect and therefore unreliable as a preventative measure. Despite this caveat, H1 blockade does seem to mitigate the severity of symptoms in a group of patients [355]. One practice is to attempt an empirical trial of H1 blockers in cases where EIA happens often or is extreme, stopping the trial if no evidence of benefit is forthcoming.

H1 blockers may be administered prn (*pro re nata*) 2 h before exercise or daily, according to how often exercise occurs. Second-generation histamine blockers, which are not sedating, e.g. cetirizine 10 mg od/bd or fexofenadine 180 mg od/bd or loratadine 10 mg od/bd are preferable, although sedation can become an issue at the higher doses of cetirizine and loratadine [382].

Other pharmacotherapy recommendations: misoprostol (a synthetic analogue of prostaglandin E1) [387, 388] and omalizumab [389] are recorded as beneficial in case reports.

Recommencing exercise routines: The general advice is to start with a low impact exercise (most likely not to provoke symptoms) and build up by stages over the course of weeks or months, simultaneously keeping clear of known co-factors [382].

Ceasing exercise immediately when symptoms begin: Patients are advised to be alert for the early warning signs (e.g. excessive fatigue, itching, spreading redness) and cease exerting themselves as soon as they occur [382].

Epinephrine: When symptoms first appear, the epinephrine auto-injector should be placed ready for use. If dizziness occurs, advise a lying position, then inject into a muscle (preferably the anterolateral portion of the thigh). If the patient is already lying down, this is preferable. No delay should occur between the onset of circulatory or breathing symptoms (e.g. being light-headed, laryngeal constriction, dyspnoea) and injection of epinephrine [382].

Patients are advised to keep the auto-injector on their person, or at least in very close proximity, on all occasions when exertion, whether exercising or other type, is likely. Caution should be given that leaving an auto-injector in a locker may result in disaster. If a previous reaction has been extreme, a second dose needs to be possible. If so required, time it for 5–15 min after first administration. The doctor should discuss methods of keeping an auto-injector to hand as bulky items can be a hindrance for certain sports, e.g. running, leading to reluctance. Talking about such issues at the outset can improve patient concordance. More recent auto-injector models are shaped and sized similarly to a mobile phone and can be carried with ease in a pocket or worn on a wristband intended for a mobile [382].

2.6.7.1 Further Precautions

EIA sufferers should not exercise alone or without constant supervision. The other person present, whether a professional or non-professional (companion, instructor, etc.), needs to be informed about the signs and symptoms related to anaphylaxis and to know how to give the auto-injector. A telephone able to dial for emergency assistance is a must [382].

A graded series of exercises of increasing impact proved beneficial in a retrospective observational study of EIA sufferers [356]. Activities that can be reliably introduced in a graded way are the ones patients should choose.

In addition, wherever it is practicable, the exercise should be of a form that permits being interrupted as required. Patients who take part in sports activities where each team member is necessary for the whole to function (such as cheerleading competitions) may ignore the advice to stop when mild symptoms appear in order not to let others down. Avoidance of this type of activity is preferable, and alternative activities must be sought, although participants in elite athletic events will likely resist the pressure to change sport after such an investment of effort to reach the top. This type of patient will need more intensive assistance with writing a care plan and might need follow-up at closer intervals [382].

Just as occurs with anaphylaxis of any cause, where possible, patients should not be taking chronic prescriptions, e.g. beta-blocking or ACEi drugs [382].

2.7 Latex Allergy

2.7.1 Introduction

Natural latex rubber (NLR) has been in large-scale use for more than one hundred years. The first mentions in English of immediate hypersensitivity to natural rubber in the literature are from 1979, and since then there has been a vast increase in such reporting [390]. A natural rubber tip used to administer barium enemas caused 16 deaths before being recalled in 1991 by the US FDA (Food and Drug Administration) [391]. The event made more people aware of type I allergy to naturally occurring rubber used in medical devices. More than 2 in 100 workers in healthcare have occupational asthma linked to NLR, and 10–17% of workers are sensitised to the substance [392].

Latex allergy is defined as allergic response to items produced from naturally occurring latex rubber. The epitopes are proteins from the rubber plant that remain after processing into products. There are also several other chemicals found in such products that arise not from the rubber plant itself but from processing. Thus for some patients, the allergen is to one of these other chemicals found within latex products. Allergologists need to differentiate between these allergy types. A hypersensitivity to chemicals raises the suspicion of a latex allergy and results in referral to dermatology for testing [393].

Having an atopic diathesis (e.g. allergic rhinitis) or being in regular contact with rubber products are the principal risk factors for the development of NLR allergy. The risk profile matches those who use NLR gloves occupationally, such as doctors, dentists, nurses and other healthcare professionals. It is frequently the case that children with chronic conditions (e.g. spina bifida) who have been repeatedly exposed to NLR products develop hypersensitivity [393].

NLR allergy can result in anaphylaxis if the sufferer comes into contact with NLR. Anaphylaxis develops minutes after being exposed and typically causes symptoms of widespread urticaria, dyspnoea, and hypotension. Since there is an associated mortality, administration of epinephrine by injection should occur without delay if symptoms begin to develop. The likelihood of an anaphylactic reaction increases when there is contact between the NLR-containing product across a breached epidermis and a mucosal surface. Such contact may occur orally (e.g. inflating balloons, dental procedures or receiving anaesthesia), vaginally (sexual intercourse with a condom, vaginal examination), with the gut (per rectum examination or enema use), or intraurethrally (e.g. when a catheter is inserted). It also happens in the course of surgery since surgeons use latex gloves in general during operations [393].

Another group whose risk of being sensitised to NLR is above average are people who have repeatedly been exposed to NLR, such as following multiple surgical procedures, particularly in childhood, as is the case with patients having a myelomeningocele (spina bifida) or correction of abnormalities in the urinary and genital systems. Here the frequency may exceed 60% [394].

The following at-risk groups have been identified [394]:

- Workers in healthcare
- Workers producing NLR
- Spina bifida sufferers or those who have had urogenital surgery for malformations
- Those with multiple or long duration operations, or who have had mucosal contact with NLR devices, the more so if in childhood
- Patients with known atopy or food allergy (cross-reactivity is highest with bananas, avocados, passion fruit, chestnuts, kiwis, melons, tomatoes, and celery).

2.7.2   NLR Products

NLR products are made from the sap of rubber trees, *Hevea brasiliensis*, that are cultivated commercially. The sap is collected and then heated in the presence of several preservative chemicals, in particular, ammonia, the purpose of which is to further improve the compound's qualities. There are a number of quite small proteins dissolved in latex, and these are the antigens to which IgE is produced in NLR allergy. There are a minimum of ten such proteins [395]. Accelerators and antioxidants that are used in the reaction may contribute substantially to the development of type IV reactions, as well as allergic and irritant contact dermatitis [394].

NLR can be manufactured by injection into moulds, or through dipping processes, the latter being employed to produce gloves, condoms, and balloons. Items manufactured by dipping or containing the softest NLR grades contain the greatest concentration of rubber proteins and thus possess the greatest allergenicity. Powdered cornstarch is put inside NLR gloves during production to ensure smoothness and prevent sticking. It has been demonstrated that particles of NLR proteins can stick to the cornstarch and be blown into the air when gloves are taken off [396].

Places with high levels of exposure, e.g. operating theatres and delivery suites, where powdered gloves are common, have enough latex floating in the air to provoke non-minor symptoms in pre-sensitised people. Different manufacturers, different production lots, and types of glove account for the variable levels of ability to provoke an allergic response. It also depends on the rebound of the NLR when stretched gloves are removed [397, 398].

2.7.3   Pathophysiology

Exposure to NLR may be associated with a trio of clinical syndromes [399]:

Irritant dermatitis is produced by physical damage to the skin as a result of gloves abrading the skin, and most NLR-related localised skin eruptions are of this kind. It does not depend on immune processes and has no allergic complications. It is therefore beyond the scope of this chapter. It may, however, be mistaken for a type IV response. Since any type of persistent inflammation of the skin of the hands amongst healthcare workers has the potential to increase susceptibility to hospital-acquired infections, amongst which are included blood-borne infections, attention needs to be paid to recognising the problem and getting rid of irritant substances [399].

A second type is the delayed (type IV) hypersensitivity response, with a characteristic allergic contact dermatitis. If a person has already been sensitised to NLR, contact with the skin or mucosae of that individual by NLR results in symptoms within a 24–48 h window. Typically, it is traces of chemical accelerators and antioxidants still present from the manufacturing stage that provoke the symptoms. Langerhans-type dendritic cells are responsible for ingesting the antigens and using the processed antigen to signal to skin T-cells.

Whilst a multitude of objects may create sensitivity, possibly the most usual for adults are nonsterile NLR gloves used for examinations and, for children, the soles of footwear. People with an allergic diathesis are more prone to type IV hypersensitivity. Eczematous reactions may then lay the ground for more sensitisation or an infection to occur [399].

The third type is the least frequently encountered, but the most serious. It is mediated through IgE specific to NLR proteins and is therefore a type I reaction. As previously observed, proteins in NLR have a high allergenicity and wide variation, arising from the manufacturing variables. IgE in sensitised individuals cross-links within mast cell and basophil membranes in response to allergen binding, and this then initiates histamine degranulation together with the secretion of other signalling molecules in the allergic pathway [399, 400].

Exposure to NLR may happen if latex is brought into proximity with skin, mucosal surfaces, or the viscera or peritoneum. Until now, the majority of sensitisations amongst adults have occurred due to powder-containing NLR examination gloves, bringing antigen into skin contact and allowing allergen inhalation. For the most part, this has affected healthcare workers wearing the gloves. Thankfully, this may be becoming less of an issue as powderless, "hypoallergenic" or non-NLR gloves are adopted in use by hospitals [401].

2.7.4 Epidemiology

The prevalence of NLR allergy in general populations is between 1 and 5%, but higher in atopy sufferers. The frequency goes up amongst groups whose jobs expose them persistently to latex [402]. Amongst healthcare staff, rates of 8–12% are observed [403] and NLR industrial workers have a rate of 10% or above. A study of emergency medical services staff showed a rate of 14%, but 54% in Accident and Emergency departments specialised in paediatric care [404–406]. Possessing an allergic diathesis makes the risk of being sensitised through work higher [399]. The highest recorded prevalence for NLR allergy was in patients with spina bifida or congenital malformations of the genitourinary tract. The rate was 20–68%. It seems that sensitisation took place as a result of having undergone many procedures on the urinary tract, rectum, and spinal cord covering in addition to repeated operations in early life. Children whose spinal cords are injured similarly have a higher rate of NLR allergy, but paediatric spinal dysraphism was associated with a low frequency in one study [408]. It may be the case that spina bifida sufferers are genetically prone to NLR sensitisation. Possession of spina bifida and the DRB and DQB1 alleles of the human leucocyte antigen was associated with a greater likelihood of generating IgE specific to a common NLR antigenic determinant. Atopy conferred an enhanced risk within this group, as with other groups [399].

There are other groups with a background of multiple operations or other procedures where NLR exposure can occur whose risk is elevated vis-à-vis the population as a whole. Those with cerebral palsy, learning disability, or paraplegia similarly have a seemingly elevated risk for NLR allergy, most likely as a result of NLR encountered repeatedly in medical settings. Having a food allergy to avocado, banana, kiwi, papaya, chestnut, nectarine, or peach increases the risk of NLR allergy. The antigens underlying cross-reactions have been identified in these cases [399].

Type I hypersensitivity predisposes to anaphylaxis and airway obstruction, which have associated mortalities. Mortality is recorded in cases where NLR-containing devices were in use during an operation or procedure. Anaphylaxis linked to NLR allergy has happened following childbirth, use of surgical equipment, intravenous injections, inflating balloons by mouth, use of condoms, and hyperbaric therapy [409–413].

2.7.5 History

When symptoms occur within minutes of contact with NLR, it is a type I (immediate) reaction, whereas a delay of up to 2 days indicates a type IV (delayed) hypersensitivity.

Symptoms for a type I reaction may involve [399]:

- Itching of skin and mucosal surfaces where contact has occurred
- Cutaneous oedema, mucosae, or subcutaneous tissue
- Dysphonia
- Watering eyes
- Difficulty breathing
- Dizziness, brief loss of consciousness
- Griping intestinal pain
- Desire to vomit or actual vomiting
- Watery stools

2.7.6 Causes

Where exposure to NLR has taken place may be evident or hidden. Patients may or may not be able to give an account of their allergy to NLR. Contact with NLR may occur via skin, mucosal surfaces, or the airways (mouth, nose, and trachea).

Both healthcare practitioners and patients run the risk of an allergic reaction during healthcare interactions if they have been sensitised to NLR. Inhaling NLR particles inadvertently is a common occurrence in clinics, where powder-carrying NLR particles becomes airborne after glove use and may stay suspended for several hours. If powderless gloves are in use, the risk diminishes. Inhaling antigen may also be a hazard outside a hospital setting, due to other NLR items lubricated with dry powder, as may the breathing in of minute pieces of tire from vehicles in heavily congested areas [399].

Amongst many possible sources of NLR, the following are frequently encountered [399]:

- Gloves (examination, surgical, and for domestic use)
- Tourniquets and blood pressure cuffs
- Stethoscopes
- Catheters
- Tubing for vascular access, associated devices, and ports; syringe drivers
- ECG and EEG pads
- Protective eyewear
- Ventilation equipment
- Surgical drains and tubing
- Tops on vials for multiple use
- Rubber dams
- Tyres
- Rubber handles
- Carpets
- Soles of footwear and elasticated portions of clothing
- Condoms, contraceptive caps
- Balloons
- Baby feeding bottles and dummies
- Erasers, computer mouse pads, and rubber bands

2.7.7   Laboratory Studies

The diagnosis of NLR allergy and management decisions are clinically determined [414]. Within Accident and Emergency, pathology results usually arrive too late to influence management. In non-emergency settings, there are several investigations of potential value. Whilst total circulating IgE levels may be raised in type I allergic response, the finding lacks both specificity and sensitivity [399].

Radioallergosorbent tests (RAST) can identify between 50 and 100% of cases with NLR-specific IgE, and between 63 and 100% of those positives are true positives. The value in prediction is dependent on which form the test takes, which group of patients is being tested and where the allergen came from. RAST has value alongside a history consistent with NLR allergy and is safe to use. As RAST testing is developing, the sensitivity and specificity are going up [415].

ELISA (enzyme-linked assay) for NLR-specific immunoglobulin E can be used in the same way [416]. To assess risk, optimise treatment, and appreciate the underlying pathological mechanisms, genomic profiling has future potential [417].

2.7.8 Management

Within clinical workplaces, managing NLR allergy has two principal aims: to stop allergy developing in the first place and to treat it in healthcare workers, and to be able to care for NLR-allergic patients safely. The main tactic is to avoid NLR contact. A high number of those with persistent contact with powder-containing gloves (the product with the highest allergenic capability) become NLR-allergic. Employers need a strategy in place to reduce the total amount of NLR exposure that occurs, such as through the use of powderless, low-protein NLR or non-NLR gloves. Newer manufacturing technologies have produced powderless gloves which can be put on more easily than the powder-containing versions. Normally powder is intended as a dry lubricant. Certain more recent glove types result in minimal amounts of soluble or airborne antigen, but brands vary greatly in this respect. Anyone with an NLR allergy should only use gloves that are not latex. The National Institute of Occupational Safety and Health (NIOSH) has recently put out advisory guidance in documentary format about the use of NLR in occupational settings. For any activity where the risk of infectious contamination is low, such as housework and cooking, or maintenance, non-NLR gloves are recommended [394, 418].

NLR within any type of product is potentially a stimulus for a reaction. As a result, a thorough check on all the products in domestic, occupational, and healthcare settings should be undertaken. More and more manufacturers are publishing checklists of products that contain NLR. Certain non-NLR products are around as strong and allow similar sensitivity to latex versions. Vinyl gloves cannot prevent viral infection as well as NLR, but the American Society for Testing and Materials (ASTM) has shown the high level of barrier integrity possible with other non-NLR materials. Vinyl's costs are similar to NLR; however, other materials typically cost more [394].

Doctors need to both advocate for and educate their NLR-allergic patients. If a healthcare employee has undergone NLR sensitisation, occupational functioning may be impossible if NLR-containing materials are not avoided and the aerosolised NLR particle count not reduced at work. Accommodating these needs does, however, in addition, mean fewer healthcare workers become newly sensitised in the future [394].

To be able to manage a case of NLR-sensitivity effectively, it is essential to distinguish between true (immediate) allergy of type I to NLR and a contact eczema brought on by irritation to the skin from other factors. If the diagnosis points towards a type I reaction, the surroundings will need to be free of NLR. Within a hospital, there need to be standard procedures applying to A and E, operating theatres, and other patient areas, where NLR exposure may take place, and documented procedures should be consultable by all employees, including housekeeping employees. When admitting a patient, the clerking should include enquiries about NLR allergy, or a questionnaire should be given. The presence of NLR allergy needs to be written in the records and displayed on the door of the patient's room, by the bed, and on an alert wristband. Non-NLR equipment should be available in A and E, operating theatres, and on the crash trolley. Hypoallergenic latex gloves still contain enough traces of antigen to provoke reactions and cannot be used near allergy sufferers [394]. If an operating list contains a patient known to be

NLR-allergic, it is better to perform the operation at the start of the list, since that is when NLR particles floating in the air should be at their lowest. If the blood pressure measuring equipment has NLR-containing elements, wrapping the patient's limbs should be done as a precaution against contact. Recommended practice has been to avoid drawing up medication through vials with rubber tops or to allow medication to rest in preloaded syringes made from NLR, nor to utilise NLR-containing ports for intravascular access. But this advice may be unnecessarily complicated unless the NLR allergy is very acute. Some doctors prescribe prophylactic histamine blockers, corticosteroids, and H_2 antagonists, yet such a practice has not prevented anaphylaxis from happening [394, 419].

2.7.8.1 Accident and Emergency Care

It is essential to keep patients seeking care for non-allergy problems, but who are known or suspected to have an NLR hypersensitivity, in an area away from latex. Included in this warning are all patients who have spina bifida [399].

Treatment of NLR allergy active reactions follow the pattern of treating generalised allergic reactions of whatever source, but with the addition of extra care to avoid inadvertent further NLR exposure, which would worsen the situation. In many cases, Accident and Emergency departments, clinics, and hospitals in general are dangerous places for sufferers of NLR allergy, the more so when there are still powdered gloves being used [399].

There needs to be access to equipment used in resuscitating patients that does not have NLR-containing items as part of it. One common way to achieve this is by having a separate, movable crash trolley with all equipment on it (intubation and ventilation equipment, etc.) checked to exclude the possibility of inadvertent NLR exposure [399].

In a more routine setting, wherever a patient's allergy presents risk, non-NLR equipment is to be preferred. Severe responses have been triggered in patients with sensitivities through per vaginam and per rectum examination done using

NLR gloves, urinary catheter insertion with an NLR-containing piece of equipment, intravenous access using ports made of NLR, and breathing in NRL particles bound to glove powder [399].

Specialists need to be observant about avoiding all NLR contact in allergic patients, both when examining patients and when conducting a procedure [399].

Patients being conveyed to investigations elsewhere need to go in ways that avoid NLR contact [399].

To be able to correctly classify a medical device as latex-free in the past took great effort as each manufacturer had to be contacted separately; however, it is now more straightforward to ensure the safety of NLR-allergic patients, since, as of 1999, the US FDA has mandated the application of warning labels on equipment containing NLR [420]. Coupled with this change, manufacturers now have multiple options for non-NLR containing materials to supply for routine and invasive use. It is worth noting, however, that labels may sometimes lack clarity and the potential for mixing up devices in busy clinical practice still exists [399].

2.7.8.2 Treatment of Severe Allergic Reactions to NLR

If anaphylaxis occurs to NLR, epinephrine should be given by the appropriate injector (EpiPen or EpiPen Jr) without delay and medical assistance sought urgently.

Generalised, acute allergic responses to NLR do not differ from other such acute responses. Following the ABC pathway, oxygen is given and epinephrine administered along with corticosteroids. Diphenhydramine (Benadryl) is helpful for hives. Whilst resuscitating, pay attention to avoid further latex exposure. Intravenous fluids and nebuliser treatment may be necessary. Go on treating by observation following symptomatic improvement. It is sadly ironic that Accident and Emergency and clinics may present special danger to those with NLR allergies. This irony may be resolved with the increasing attention paid to the significant risks to health that NLR allergies present [394].

2.8 Idiopathic Anaphylaxis

2.8.1 Background

Idiopathic anaphylaxis (IA) is a well-characterised syndrome in which anaphylaxis occurs in the absence of an identifiable precipitant. Such cases have identical symptomatology with other varieties of anaphylaxis. Attacks occur at unpredictable intervals, and some have been reported as leading to death of the patient [422].

Bacal et al. were the first to write about IA (in 1978), using the label for a group of 11 cases in which an anaphylactic response could not be accounted for [423]. This case series has since been enlarged to encompass more than 335 cases. The frequency of allergic diathesis in the series was reported as 48%, reflecting the same percentage amongst the original cases, which were all from Spain.

It is frequently the case that anaphylaxis can be linked to a definite antigenic substance, e.g. foodstuffs, drugs, or insect venom. The diagnosis of IA is possible when no antigen can be identified after a suitable investigation, and there is no other condition present, like mastocytosis, which could better account for the symptoms [422].

IA is a diagnosis only made when other diagnoses have been excluded and should only be offered after a very careful history has been taken, physical examination performed, and past medical history checked out. Laboratory investigations may help to exclude particular antigens and the multitude of disorders which can mimic IA. A detailed and comprehensive history in all likelihood will form the backbone of clinical evaluation, since the tests chosen will depend on the history. The account should home in on the circumstances pertaining at the time of each anaphylactic reaction, how often the reactions occur and with what severity, how treatment affected the symptoms, objective signs as recorded to substantiate the anaphylaxis, and the chance that an episode was actually triggered by a specific allergen.

For IA to be diagnosed, the following established causes of anaphylaxis need to be ruled out: foodstuffs, drugs, insect venom, latex rubber, contrast agents used in radiology, and exercise [425].

Allergic reactions to food occur at a probable frequency of 1–2% of the general population and are the most frequent reason for anaphylaxis [426]. Mostly, symptoms start 5 min to half an hour after eating, sometimes after 1 or 2 h, but seldom after that. Symptoms beginning many hours post food should point to different diagnostic possibilities, as should the fact that the patient has subsequently tolerated the same food. Shellfish, fish, groundnuts, milk, eggs, soya, and wheat allergies together make up 90% of the food allergies seen. Food allergy diagnoses can be verified through cutaneous tests and, at times, doubly blinded formal food challenge [425].

2.8.2   Epidemiology

IA counts amongst the most frequent reasons for anaphylaxis. In a retrospective study, around one in three cases of anaphylaxis were of this type [427]. Estimates put the number of affected people, just within the USA, at 30,000 [422].

IA is more frequent in adults, albeit also occurring in children [428–430]. In a number of case series, approaching 70% of IA sufferers were female, and around 50% had atopy [428, 432, 433]. A diagnosis of IA does not exclude comorbidity with other forms of anaphylaxis, e.g. due to food, drugs, and exercising [428]. Within the USA, a prevalence of 1 in 10,000 has been reported for IA [433].

2.8.3   Pathogenesis

Both anaphylaxis of known cause and IA feature enhanced activity by mast cells. In addition, IA is associated with increased lymphocytic activity, although why this should be the case remains unclear [424].

2.8.3.1   Mast Cell Activation

The levels of mast cell mediators in IA patients are raised in an acute episode. This includes histamine in blood and urine [430], and circulating total tryptase [430, 434]. By contrast, total tryptase is persistently raised in mastocytosis, even when symptoms have resolved [435–437]. A subset of patients with IA who have a clonal mast cell proliferation following a mutation in c-KIT has been identified from one study. This diagnosis needs excluding before pressing ahead with the diagnosis of IA [437].

2.8.3.2   Lymphocyte and Basophil Activation

During the acute phases, IA patients have higher numbers of activated T-cells in the circulation than occur in the periods of remission. Their activated B-cell numbers are also higher, in both phases of the disorder, than in normal controls or in cases of chronic idiopathic urticaria [438]. Microarray analysis has revealed that cells taken from IA patients express differentially certain genes associated with CD203c production. CD203c is a definite indicator of basophil activation [439].

2.8.4   Diagnosis

IA can only be diagnosed where other competing diagnoses have been excluded through a process of meticulous history taking and physical examination. Cutaneous tests, RAST, and other laboratory investigations are generally needed to exclude specific allergens as triggers and the several other disorders outlined below which can mimic IA. As with all allergic diagnoses, the patient's account is of central importance in dictating what tests will follow on [422]. Levels of serum tryptase (secreted by mast cells) are highly valuable to differentiate anaphylaxis from the multiple anaphylaxis mimics [440].

A range of tests to confirm or disconfirm a putative allergen may be performed, amongst which might feature: cutaneous and laboratory-based testing for specific IgE to various foods and medications, IgE to alpha-gal, blood tryptase in acute episodes and at baseline, 24 h urine collection to test for the metabolites of histamine, prostaglandin D2 in urine, and peripheral blood to test for mutated D816V. Food challenge and, in certain circumstance, bone marrow biopsy may be helpful. Sometimes, fresh foods used for prick tests may give a more reliable (i.e. possessing greater sensitivity) result than commercially prepared extracts [441, 442].

New insights are altering the way clinicians use the laboratory to investigate the true nature of the allergen. Such insights include the role played by carbohydrate determinants and alpha-gal [443, 444], and ascertaining how important mastocytosis and mast cell activating disorders are as reasons for anaphylaxis [442, 445, 446].

2.8.5 Differential Diagnosis

1. **Established triggers for immediate systemic reactions** [422]

   (a) **Modulated through immunoglobulin E**
       Allergy to foodstuffs is the most frequently found reason for anaphylaxis and its frequency is 1–2% in the population. The onset of symptoms is usually between 5 and 30 min following exposure, at times 1–2 h later, but seldom longer than that. Symptoms that commence more than a few hours after eating should encourage the doctor to question the diagnosis, as should the situation where the patient has managed to eat the putative allergen on a later occasion without problems. Milk, eggs, groundnuts, tree nuts, fish, shellfish, soya, and wheat are the most frequently encountered types of food allergy, collectively accounting for about 90% of allergies of this type. Allergies to mustard and certain other spices are frequently misdiagnosed as IA.

Medications not infrequently also trigger anaphylactic actions. When taking the history, pay careful attention to prescribed medications, dietary supplements, herbal medicines (Bee pollen, Echinacea) and OTC medicines, particularly aspirin and the NSAIDs [422].

(b) **Exercise-induced anaphylaxis** [422]
(c) **Food-dependent, exercise-induced anaphylaxis** [422]
(d) **Drug reactions not mediated through IgE** [422]

- Aspirin and NSAIDs
- Opiate painkillers
- Angiotensin-converting enzyme inhibitors (ACE inhibitors)
- Contrast agents used in radiology

2. **Asthma that mimics IA**
3. **Systemic mastocytosis**
4. **Hereditary angioedema**
5. **Munchausen's syndrome (factitious stridor or symptoms of anaphylaxis)**
6. **Undifferentiated somatoform idiopathic anaphylaxis**
7. **Miscellaneous diagnoses**

(a) Panic disorder
(b) Globus sensation
(c) Histamine-rich food flushing

2.8.5.1 Exercise-Induced Anaphylaxis (EIA)

Exercise-induced anaphylaxis is likely to be one of the most common conditions misdiagnosed as IA. The aetiology involves the activation of mastocytes as a result of exercising. In exercise-induced anaphylaxis, there is pruritus over the whole body, hives, angioedema, gut pain, loose stools, and syncope as a result of extreme low blood pressure. Diagnosing the condition can be tricky since the reaction does not invariably follow on from exercising. Elite athletes are frequently amongst this group. A case series involving 266 patients, all of whom had anaphylaxis, ascertained that 19 (7.1%) had exercise-induced anaphylaxis. For anaphylaxis to occur in conjunction with exercise, a subgroup of EIA patients must have consumed particular foodstuffs (often wheat) within a 2 h window prior to exercising. This variant is termed food-related, exercise-induced anaphylaxis (FDEIA) [422].

Whilst hereditary angioedema may superficially resemble idiopathic anaphylaxis, the absence of urticaria or the symptomatology associated with anaphylaxis, the slow progression of the angioedematous element, which is associated with considerable pain, and the lack of itching should alert the clinician to the mimicry. Knowing that other members of the family have the disorder makes it easier to diagnose, but a negative family history does not exclude the disorder.

Dental surgery may cause a flare-up, as may a number of other sources of minor trauma. Diagnosing the disorder is vital, since potentially fatal reactions may not be stopped by epinephrine administration, whilst androgens (danazol, stanozolol) may be of use in prevention.

Low levels of complement proteins and C1 esterase inhibitor or reduced C1 esterase activity supports the diagnosis of IA [422].

2.8.5.2   Systemic Mastocytosis

Systemic mastocytosis is an uncommon disorder. Patients have attacks wherein their skin abruptly reddens and is accompanied by pruritus, there is urticaria, abdominodynia, and, on occasion, lowered blood pressure. Greater than 50% of such patients possess "freckles" which respond to rubbing by becoming hives. The systemic consequences include infiltration by mast cells of the bone marrow, resulting in osteoporosis or ongoing scarring. Cases may also develop peptic ulceration, hepatomegaly, loose and watery stools, debility, and weight loss.

Mast cell tryptase in serum typically remains high intraepisodically, with a rise following an acute episode. Bone scanning may also be of assistance in diagnosing cases.

It may be tricky to differentiate between an initial asthma episode and constriction of the bronchi occurring within the setting of IA. An asthma episode will be different from IA, however, in lacking signs of a generalised anaphylactic reaction [422].

2.8.5.3   Munchausen's Stridor/Anaphylaxis

Stridor in Munchausen's involves an apparent abrupt onset of dyspnoea together with loud breathing sounds emanating from the neck. This is a factitious disorder. Munchausen's syndrome patients deliberately set in motion anaphylaxis by ingesting known allergenic foods. A possible presentation would be a case of known groundnut allergy knowingly ingesting peanut before ringing for an ambulance [422].

2.8.5.4   Undifferentiated Somatoform Idiopathic Anaphylaxis (US-IA)

This is a variety of IA wherein objective signs that confirm anaphylaxis are not present. Cases give a history of lightheadedness, syncope, laryngeal constriction, urticaria, and being short of breath. Despite this, objective observations of an acute attack which could substantiate the diagnosis are not available [422].

2.8.6   Treatment

Discussion of the treatment for IA can be usefully considered under the headings "acute intervention" and "long-term prophylaxis" [424].

Interventional RCTs concerning acute intervention or long-term prophylaxis have not yet been performed. Acute intervention guidelines are founded upon experience gained by animal models of anaphylaxis, human prospective trials where anaphylaxis was or was not currently being experienced by the patient, information gleaned from observational studies, case reports of anaphylactic reactions in patients, and clinical experience [424].

Acute management: Emergency interventions in IA do not differ from the approach used in other types of anaphylaxis [424].

Epinephrine is the mainstay of acute pharmacotherapy in anaphylaxis. No other agent on its own can match epinephrine for halting the pathophysiological changes underlying anaphylaxis. There is no other medication that can stop or ameliorate oedema within the larynx and prevent circulatory failure. Time after time it has been shown that giving epinephrine too late in anaphylaxis results in a fatal outcome [447–450]. Treating anaphylaxis acutely is addressed in a separate chapter of this book.

Long-term management: Attacks of idiopathic anaphylaxis gradually decrease in frequency as time goes on. Guidelines depend for their evidence upon observational studies, case reporting, and practical experience [424].

How the disorder is managed in the long-term hinges upon how frequently episodes occur [430, 451]:

- Pharmacotherapy for frequent attacks may necessitate a combination of oral steroid (prednisolone) and an H1 blocker, typically lasting 3 months.
- Pharmacotherapy for infrequent attacks is usually not recommended.

2.8.6.1 Combination Therapy with Glucocorticoids and Antihistamines

Prophylactic pharmacotherapy aimed at the prevention of recurrence is generally needed for cases where episodes occur frequently, despite the fact that a proportion of such cases spontaneously improve even in the absence of glucocorticoid treatment [452]. The evidence for combining glucocorticoid and H1 blocker drugs comes from case reports and observational research [428, 451]. There are no studies addressing glucocorticoid use on its own, as an H1 blocker has invariably been co-prescribed. To illustrate this point, in one particular case series, 22 cases received prednisolone and hydroxyzine, and a subgroup in addition received a sympathomimetic by mouth [430]. Of the 22 participants, 19 suffered fewer relapses following the beginning of treatment. Once the treatment course was finished, around half the patients were in remission (in other words, asymptomatic despite the absence of steroid treatment in the previous 12 months). A proportion of these patients continued to take a H1 blocker [424].

It is possible to combine a steroid and histamine blocker when an attack has just occurred or immediately upon reaching the diagnosis [424]:

- Prednisolone: Typically a trial of prednisolone begins with the dose of 40–60 mg by mouth daily continuing for 7 days or up to the point where symptoms have stopped. The dose can be continued *alt die* for 14 days or longer. Reduce the dose to 5–10 mg *alt die* for 2 weeks, as long as no symptoms emerge. Typically 1 week of treatment is enough to prevent episodes [430]. Whilst decreasing the dosage, if symptoms start to emerge, prednisolone will need to be increased. Having achieved symptomatic control, the prescriber can then reduce the dose once more. If again during this second reduction symptoms reappear, consideration is given to using additional medications [424].
- H1 blocker: H1 blockade is normally prescribed alongside steroid treatment. Trial evidence only covers the first generation of histamine blockers in the treatment of IA, but in clinical practice, second-generation antihistamines, e.g. cetirizine, at a dosage of 10 mg o.d. by mouth, are usually preferable since they offer greater benefit for the same risk. It is usual to continue the H1 blocker following stoppage of the glucocorticoid, particularly in patients with advanced age or who have previously had extreme reactions, or suffer from other illnesses at the same time [424].

Alternative therapeutic possibilities: There is some evidence available from case reports and small-scale case series to support the use of alternative medications [422].

- Ketotifen acts as an H1 blocker and stabilises mast cell degranulation but can be over-sedating. Its use in oral form is not licensed within the USA, nor is it licensed in several other countries. Typically ketotifen is at a dose of 2 mg by mouth b.d. or t.d.s. [428, 453].
- Sodium cromoglycate by mouth and leukotriene antagonists, for example montelukast, are documented as having clinical benefits in certain cases [428, 430].

Glucocorticoid-dependent idiopathic anaphylaxis: Amongst patients who have frequent bouts of IA, 20% experience symptoms as a result of withdrawing prednisolone. This situation is described as glucocorticoid-dependent IA. Idiopathic anaphylaxis which does not respond to the typical therapeutic regimens is termed "malignant". According to one researcher, the threshold for referring to the disorder as "malignant" is when prednisolone needs to be titrated to at least 20 mg o.d. or 60 mg *alt die* to gain symptom control [430].

Managing symptoms which do not respond to therapy: In spite of therapeutic intervention as described above, there remains a group of patients whose symptoms are not under control or who experience recurrence when prednisolone is withdrawn. There are some case reports indicative of success where omalizumab or rituximab have been employed in these situations [424].

Omalizumab: This is a monoclonal-type antibody with a specificity for IgE. Its efficacy has been demonstrated in a case where both food-related anaphylaxis and IA had previously occurred [454]. A separate case report detailed how symptomatic control was achieved in a case suffering from both IA and severe allergic asthma [455]. Dosage and side effects of omalizumab are discussed elsewhere.

Rituximab: There is one case report in which an individual suffering from severe idiopathic anaphylaxis, which had not responded to H1 blockade, leukotriene antagonists, systemic steroid treatment, or dietary restriction lasting 3 years and affecting three separate potential triggers to allergy, received omalizumab for 8 months empirically [456]. The anaphylactic attacks, which had been occurring on a weekly basis, were brought to an end by the administration of rituximab 1000 mg intravenously on two occasions separated by a 14-day interval. Following the second administration, there was a period of 9 months in which no anaphylactic episode occurred. Episodes restarted when B-cell levels returned to normal. Treatment continued as a reduced dose at 6 monthly intervals [424].

Relative contraindications to particular medications: Where practicable, avoid the use of beta-blockers in cases of idiopathic anaphylaxis given that they may hinder the action of epinephrine [430]. The ongoing treatment and management of patients with known anaphylaxis is discussed elsewhere [424].

References

1. Sampson HA, Aceves S, Bock SA, James J, Jones S, et al. Food allergy: a practice parameter update-2014. J Allergy Clin Immunol. 2014;134(5):1016–25.
2. Sicherer SC. Food allergies. In: Kaliner MA, editor. Medscape. http://emedicine.medscape.com/article/135959-overview. Accessed 26 June 2016.
3. Bock SA, Munoz-Furlong A, Sampson HA. Further fatalities caused by anaphylactic reactions to food, 2001-2006. J Allergy Clin Immunol. 2007;119(4):1016–8.
4. Food allergy: a practice parameter. Ann Allergy Asthma Immunol. 2006;96(Suppl):S1–68.
5. Rona RJ, et al. The prevalence of food allergy: a meta-analysis. J Allergy Clin Immunol. 2007;120:638–46.
6. Sicherer SH, Sampson HA. Peanut allergy: emerging concepts and approaches for an apparent epidemic. J Allergy Clin Immunol. 2007;120:491–503. quiz 504–505.
7. Boden SR, Burks AW. Anaphylaxis: a history with emphasis on food allergy. Immunol Rev. 2011;242(1):247–57.
8. Sampson HA, Burks AW. Adverse reactions to foods. In: Adkinson Jr NF, Bochner BS, Busse WW, Holgate ST, Lemanske Jr RF, Simons FER, editors. Middleton's allergy: principles and practice. 7th ed. St Louis: Mosby; 2009. p. 1139–67.

9. Anonymous. The food allergy and anaphylaxis management act of 2009. Senate Bill 456, introduced into the United States Senate. http://thomas.loc.gov. Accessed 20 Oct 2009.

10. Elberink JNO. Significance and rationale of studies of health-related quality of life in anaphylactic disorders. Curr Opin Allergy Clin Immunol. 2006;6:298–302.

11. Herbert LJ, Dahlquist LM. Perceived history of anaphylaxis and parental overprotection, autonomy, anxiety, and depression in food allergic young adults. J Clin Psychol Med Settings. 2008;15:261–9.

12. Pieretti MM, Chung D, Pacenza R, Slotkin T, Sicherer SH. Audit of manufactured products: use of allergen advisory labels and identification of labeling ambiguities. J Allergy Clin Immunol. 2009;124:337–41.

13. Boyano-Martinez T, Garcia-Ara C, Pedrosa M, Diaz-Pena JM, Quirce S. Accidental allergic reactions in children allergic to cow's milk proteins. J Allergy Clin Immunol. 2009;123:883–8.

14. Ko J, Lee JI, Munoz-Furlong A, Li X, Sicherer SH. Use of complementary and alternative medicine by food-allergic patients. Ann Allergy Asthma Immunol. 2006;97:365–9.

15. Simons FE. Anaphylaxis. J Allergy Clin Immunol. 2010;125(2 Suppl 2):S161–81.

16. Cummings AJ, et al. The psychosocial impact of food allergy and food hypersensitivity in children, adolescents and their families: a review. Allergy. 2010;65:933–45.

17. Savage JH, et al. The natural history of egg allergy. J Allergy Clin Immunol. 2007;120:1413–147.

18. Skripak JM, et al. The natural history of IgE-mediated cow's milk allergy. J Allergy Clin Immunol. 2007;120:1172–7.

19. Bindslev-Jensen C, et al. Standardization of food challenges in patients with immediate reactions to foods—position paper from the European Academy of Allergology and Clinical Immunology. Allergy. 2004;59:690–7.

20. Bock SA, et al. Double-blind, placebo-controlled food challenge (DBPCFC) as an office procedure: a manual. J Allergy Clin Immunol. 1988;82:986–97.

21. Worth A, Nurmatov U, Sheikh A. Key components of anaphylaxis management plans: consensus findings from a national electronic Delphi study. JRSM Short Rep. 2010;1:42.

22. Sloan AE, Powers ME. A perspective on popular perceptions of adverse reactions to foods. J Allergy Clin Immunol. 1986;78(1 Pt 2):127–33.

23. Altman DR, Chiaramonte LT. Public perception of food allergy. J Allergy Clin Immunol. 1996;97(6):1247–51.

24. Rona RJ, Keil T, Summers C, Gislason D, Zuidmeer L, Sodergren E, et al. The prevalence of food allergy: a meta-analysis. J Allergy Clin Immunol. 2007;120(3):638–46.

25. Zuidmeer L, Goldhahn K, Rona RJ, Gislason D, Madsen C, Summers C, et al. The prevalence of plant food allergies: a systematic review. J Allergy Clin Immunol. 2008;121(5):1210–1218.e4.

26. Sicherer SH, Munoz-Furlong A, Sampson HA. Prevalence of peanut and tree nut allergy in the United States determined by means of a random digit dial telephone survey: a 5-year follow-up study. J Allergy Clin Immunol. 2003;112(6):1203–7.

27. Sicherer SH, Sampson HA. Food allergy. J Allergy Clin Immunol. 2010;125(2 Suppl 2):S116–25.

28. Sicherer SH. Epidemiology of food allergy. J Allergy Clin Immunol. 2011;127(3):594–602.

29. Grundy J, Matthews S, Bateman B, Dean T, Arshad SH. Rising prevalence of allergy to peanut in children: data from 2 sequential cohorts. J Allergy Clin Immunol. 2002;110(5):784–9.

30. Kagan RS, Joseph L, Dufresne C, Gray-Donald K, Turnbull E, Pierre YS, et al. Prevalence of peanut allergy in primary-school children in Montreal, Canada. J Allergy Clin Immunol. 2003;112(6):1223–8.

31. Hourihane JO, Aiken R, Briggs R, Gudgeon LA, Grimshaw KE, DunnGalvin A, et al. The impact of government advice to pregnant mothers regarding peanut avoidance on the prevalence of peanut allergy in United Kingdom children at school entry. J Allergy Clin Immunol. 2007;119(5):1197–202.

32. Jackson KD, Howie LD, Akinbami LJ. Trends in allergic conditions among children: United States, 1997–2011. U.S. Department of Health and Human Services. 2013. http://www.cdc.gov/nchs/data/databriefs/db121.pdf.

33. Weber RW. Food additives and allergy. Ann Allergy. 1993;70(3):183–90.

34. Chehade M, Mayer L. Oral tolerance and its relation to food hypersensitivities. J Allergy Clin Immunol. 2005;115(1):3–12; quiz 13.

35. Vickery BP, Scurlock AM, Jones SM, Burks AW. Mechanisms of immune tolerance relevant to food allergy. J Allergy Clin Immunol. 2011;127(3):576–84.

36. Lack G. Update on risk factors for food allergy. J Allergy Clin Immunol. 2012;129(5):1187–97.

37. Berin MC. Immunopathophysiology of food protein-induced enterocolitis syndrome. J Allergy Clin Immunol. 2015;135(5):1108–13.

38. Abernathy-Carver KJ, Sampson HA, Picker LJ, Leung DY. Milk-induced eczema is associated with the expansion of T cells expressing cutaneous lymphocyte antigen. J Clin Invest. 1995;95(2):913–8.

39. Types of allergies, food allergy. American College of Allergy, Asthma & Immunology. http://acaai.org/allergies/types/food-allergies. Accessed 26 June 2016.

40. Niggemann B, Beyer K. Factors augmenting allergic reactions. Allergy. 2014;69(12):1582–7.
41. Sicherer SH. Clinical implications of cross-reactive food allergens. J Allergy Clin Immunol. 2001;108(6):881–90.
42. Commins SP, James HR, Stevens W, Pochan SL, Land MH, King C, et al. Delayed clinical and ex vivo response to mammalian meat in patients with IgE to galactose-alpha-1,3-galactose. J Allergy Clin Immunol. 2014;134(1):108–15.
43. Bock SA, Munoz-Furlong A, Sampson HA. Fatalities due to anaphylactic reactions to foods. J Allergy Clin Immunol. 2001;107(1):191–3.
44. Varshney P, Steele PH, Vickery BP, Bird JA, Thyagarajan A, Scurlock AM, et al. Adverse reactions during peanut oral immunotherapy home dosing. J Allergy Clin Immunol. 2009;124:1351–2.
45. Sicherer SH, Sampson HA. Food allergy: recent advances in pathophysiology and treatment. Ann Rev Med. 2009;60:261–77.
46. Burks AW, Laubach S, Jones SM. Oral tolerance, food allergy, and immunotherapy: implications for future treatment. J Allergy Clin Immunol. 2008;121:1344–50.
47. Wood RA. Food-specific immunotherapy: past, present, and future. J Allergy Clin Immunol. 2008;121:336–7.
48. Plaut M, Sawyer RT, Fenton MJ. Summary of the 2008 National Institute of Allergy and Infectious Diseases-US Food and Drug Administration workshop on food allergy clinical trial design. J Allergy Clin Immunol. 2009;124:671–8.
49. Skripak JM, Nash SD, Rowley H, Brereton NH, Oh S, Hamilton RG, et al. A randomized, double-blind, placebo-controlled study of milk oral immunotherapy for cow's milk allergy. J Allergy Clin Immunol. 2008;122:1154–60.
50. Narisety SD, Skripak JM, Steele P, Hamilton RG, Matsui EC, Burks AW, et al. Open-label maintenance after milk oral immunotherapy for IgE-mediated cow's milk allergy. J Allergy Clin Immunol. 2009;124:610–2.
51. Longo G, Barbi E, Berti I, Meneghetti R, Pittalis A, Ronfani L, et al. Specific oral tolerance induction in children with very severe cow's milk-induced reactions. J Allergy Clin Immunol. 2008;121:343–7.
52. Jones SM, Pons L, Roberts JL, Scurlock AM, Perry TT, Kulis M, et al. Clinical efficacy and immune regulation with peanut oral immunotherapy. J Allergy Clin Immunol. 2009;124:292–300.
53. Hofmann AM, Scurlock AM, Jones SM, Palmer KP, Lokhnygina Y, Steele PH, et al. Safety of a peanut oral immunotherapy protocol in children with peanut allergy. J Allergy Clin Immunol. 2009;124:286–91.
54. Srivastava KD, Qu C, Zhang T, Goldfarb J, Sampson HA, Li XM. Food Allergy Herbal Formula-2 silences peanut-induced ana-

phylaxis for a prolonged posttreatment period via IFN-gamma-producing CD8+T cells. J Allergy Clin Immunol. 2009;123:443–51.

55. Leung DYM, Sampson HA, Yunginger JW, Burks AW Jr, Schneider LC, Wortel CH, et al. Effect of anti-IgE therapy in patients with peanut allergy. N Engl J Med. 2003;348:986–93.

56. Fleischer DM, Burks AW, Vickery BP, Scurlock AM, Wood RA, Jones SM, et al. Sublingual immunotherapy for peanut allergy: a randomized, double-blind, placebo-controlled multicenter trial. J Allergy Clin Immunol. 2013;131(1):119–27.e1–7.

57. Jones SM, Burks AW, Dupont C. State of the art on food allergen immunotherapy: oral, sublingual, and epicutaneous. J Allergy Clin Immunol. 2014;133(2):318–23.

58. Bollinger ME, et al. The impact of food allergy on the daily activities of children and their families. Ann Allergy Asthma Immunol. 2006;96:415–21.

59. Primeau MN, et al. The psychological burden of peanut allergy as perceived by adults with peanut allergy and the parents of peanut-allergic children. Clin Exp Allergy. 2000;30:1135–43.

60. Avery NJ, et al. Assessment of quality of life in children with peanut allergy. Pediatr Allergy Immunol. 2003;14:378–82.

61. Sheikh A, Alves B. Hospital admissions for acute anaphylaxis: time trend study. BMJ. 2000;320:1441.

62. Wood RA. The natural history of food allergy. Pediatrics. 2003;111(6 Pt 3):1631–7.

63. Skripak JM, Matsui EC, Mudd K, Wood RA. The natural history of IgE-mediated cow's milk allergy. J Allergy Clin Immunol. 2007;120(5):1172–7.

64. Savage JH, Matsui EC, Skripak JM, Wood RA. The natural history of egg allergy. J Allergy Clin Immunol. 2007;120(6):1413–7.

65. Savage JH, Kaeding AJ, Matsui EC, Wood RA. The natural history of soy allergy. J Allergy Clin Immunol. 2010;125(3):683–6.

66. Mehr S, Kakakios A, Frith K, Kemp AS. Food protein-induced enterocolitis syndrome: 16-year experience. Pediatrics. 2009;123(3):e459–64.

67. Assa'ad AH, Putnam PE, Collins MH, Akers RM, Jameson SC, Kirby CL, et al. Pediatric patients with eosinophilic esophagitis: an 8-year follow-up. J Allergy Clin Immunol. 2007;119(3):731–8.

68. National Clinical Guideline Centre. NICE clinical guideline 183, Drug allergy, Diagnosis and management of drug allergy in adults, children and young people. Methods, evidence and recommendations. 2014. https://www.nice.org.uk/guidance/cg183/evidence/drug-allergy-full-guideline-193159693. Accessed 27 June 2016.

69. Thong BY, Tan TC. Epidemiology and risk factors for drug allergy. Br J Clin Pharmacol. 2011;71(5):684–700. https://doi.org/10.1111/j.1365-2125.2010.03774.x.
70. Johansson SG, Bieber T, Dahl R, Friedmann PS, Lanier BQ, Lockey RF, et al. Revised nomenclature for allergy for global use: report of the nomenclature review committee of the World Allergy Organization, October 2003. J Allergy Clin Immunol. 2004;113:832–6.
71. World Health Organization. International drug monitoring: the role of national centres. World Health Organ Tech Rep Ser. 1972;498:1–25.
72. Rawlins MD, Thompson JV. Pathogenesis of adverse drug reactions. In: Davies DM, editor. Textbook of adverse drug reactions. Oxford: Oxford University Press; 1977. p. 10.
73. Bastuji-Garin S, Rzany B, Stern RS, Shear NH, Naldi L, Roujeau JC. Clinical classification of cases of toxic epidermal necrolysis, Stevens-Johnson syndrome, and erythema multiforme. Arch Dermatol. 1993;129:92–6.
74. Guillaume JC, Rojeau JC, Revuz J, Penso D, Touraine R. The culprit drugs in 87 cases of toxic epidermal necrolysis (Lyell's syndrome). Arch Dermatol. 1987;123:1166–70.
75. Rzany B, Hering O, Mockenhaupt M, Schröder W, Goerttler E, Ring J, Schöpf E. Histopathological and epidemiological characteristics of patients with erythema exudativum multiforme major, Stevens-Johnson syndrome and toxic epidermal necrolysis. Br J Dermatol. 1996;135:6–11.
76. French LE. Toxic epidermal necrolysis and Stevens Johnson syndrome: our current understanding. Allergol Int. 2006;55:9–16.
77. Borchers AT, Lee JL, Naguwa SM, Cheema GS, Gershwin ME. Stevens-Johnson syndrome and toxic epidermal necrolysis. Autoimmun Rev. 2008;7:598–605.
78. Shiohara T, Inaoka M, Kano Y. Drug-induced hypersensitivity syndrome (DIHS): a reaction induced by a complex interplay among herpes viruses and antiviral and antidrug immune responses. Allergol Int. 2006;55:1–8.
79. Sidoroff A, Halevy S, Bavinck JN, Vaillant L, Roujeau JC. Acute generalized exanthematous pustulosis (AGEP)—a clinical reaction pattern. J Cutan Pathol. 2001;28:113–9.
80. Halevy S. Acute generalized exanthematous pustulosis. Curr Opin Allergy Clin Immunol. 2009;9:322–8.
81. Morimoto T, Gandhi TK, Seger AC, Hsieh TC, Bates DW. Adverse drug events and medication errors: detection and classification methods. Qual Saf Health Care. 2004;13:306–14.
82. Sampson HA, Muñoz-Furlong A, Campbell RL, Adkinson NF Jr, Bock SA, Branum A, et al. Second symposium on the definition and management of anaphylaxis: summary report—Second

National Institute of Allergy and Infectious Disease/Food Allergy and Anaphylaxis Network Symposium. J Allergy Clin Immunol. 2006;117:391–7.

83. Lieberman P. Epidemiology of anaphylaxis. Curr Opin Allergy Clin Immunol. 2008;8:316–20.

84. Joint Task Force on Practice Parameters; American Academy of Allergy, Asthma and Immunology; American College of Allergy, Asthma and Immunology; Joint Council of Allergy, Asthma and Immunology, et al. Ann Allergy Asthma Immunol. 2010;105(4):259–73. https://doi.org/10.1016/j.anai.2010.08.002.

85. Pichler WJ. Delayed drug hypersensitivity reactions. Ann Intern Med. 2003;139:683–93.

86. Schmid DA, Depta JP, Luthi M, et al. Transfection of drug-specific T-cell receptors into hybridoma cells: tools to monitor drug interaction with T-cell receptors and evaluate cross-reactivity to related compounds. Mol Pharmacol. 2006;70:356–65.

87. Sieben S, Kawakubo Y, Al Masaoudi T, et al. Delayed-type hypersensitivity reaction to p-phenylenediamine is mediated by two different pathways of antigen recognition by specific alpha-beta human T-cell clones. J Allergy Clin Immunol. 2002;109:1005–11.

88. Demoly P, Viola M, Gomes ER, Romano A. Epidemiology and causes of drug hypersensitivity. In: Pichler WJ, editor. Drug hypersensitivity. Basel: Karger; 2007. p. 2–17.

89. Mockenhaupt M. Epidemiology and causes of severe cutaneous adverse reactions to drugs. In: Pichler WJ, editor. Drug hypersensitivity. Basel: Karger; 2007. p. 18–31.

90. Bousquet PJ, Demoly P, Romano A, Aberer W, Bircher A, Blanca M, et al. Pharmacovigilance of drug allergy and hypersensitivity using the ENDA-DAHD database and the GALEN platform. The Galenda project. Allergy. 2009;64:194–203.

91. Demoly P, Kropf R, Bircher A, Pichler WJ. Drug hypersensitivity: questionnaire. EAACI interest group on drug hypersensitivity. Allergy. 1999;54:999–1003.

92. Torres MJ, Blanca M, Fernandez J, Romano A, Weck A, Aberer W, Brockow K, Pichler WJ, Demoly P, ENDA, EAACI Interest Group on Drug Hypersensitivity. Diagnosis of immediate allergic reactions to beta-lactam antibiotics. Allergy. 2003;58:961–72.

93. Romano A, Blanca M, Torres MJ, Bircher A, Aberer W, Brockow K, Pichler WJ, Demoly P, ENDA, EAACI. Diagnosis of non-immediate reactions to beta-lactam antibiotics. Allergy. 2004;59:1153–60.

94. Aberer W, Bircher A, Romano A, Blanca M, Campi P, Fernandez J, Brockow K, Pichler WJ, Demoly P, European Network for Drug Allergy (ENDA), EAACI Interest Group on Drug Hypersensitivity. Drug provocation testing in the diagnosis of drug hypersensitivity reactions: general considerations. Allergy. 2003;58:854–63.

95. Moore TJ, Cohen MR, Furberg CD. Serious adverse drug events reported to the Food and Drug Administration, 1998-2005. Arch Intern Med. 2007;167(16):1752–9.

96. Kerr JR. Penicillin allergy: a study of incidence as reported by patients. Br J Clin Pract. 1994;48(1):5–7.

97. Dona I, Blanca-Lopez N, Cornejo-Garcia JA, Torres MJ, Laguna JJ, Fernandez J, et al. Characteristics of subjects experiencing hypersensitivity to non-steroidal anti-inflammatory drugs: patterns of response. Clin Exp Allergy. 2011;41(1):86–95.

98. Hedman J, Kaprio J, Poussa T, Nieminen MM. Prevalence of asthma, aspirin intolerance, nasal polyposis and chronic obstructive pulmonary disease in a population-based study. Int J Epidemiol. 1999;28(4):717–22.

99. Lee CE, Zembower TR, Fotis MA, Postelnick MJ, Greenberger PA, Peterson LR, et al. The incidence of antimicrobial allergies in hospitalized patients: implications regarding prescribing patterns and emerging bacterial resistance. Arch Intern Med. 2000;160(18):2819–22.

100. Macy EM, Contreras R. Healthcare utilization and serious infection prevalence associated with penicillin "allergy" in hospitalized patients: a cohort study. J Allergy Clin Immunol. 2014;133(2):AB153.

101. Martinez JA, Ruthazer R, Hansjosten K, Barefoot L, Snydman DR. Role of environmental contamination as a risk factor for acquisition of vancomycin-resistant enterococci in patients treated in a medical intensive care unit. Arch Intern Med. 2003;163(16):1905–12.

102. Kasper L, Sladek K, Duplaga M, Bochenek G, Liebhart J, Gladysz U, et al. Prevalence of asthma with aspirin hypersensitivity in the adult population of Poland. Allergy. 2003;58(10):1064–6.

103. Doeglas HM. Reactions to aspirin and food additives in patients with chronic urticaria, including the physical urticarias. Br J Dermatol. 1975;93(2):135–44.

104. Moore-Robinson M, Warin RP. Effect of salicylates in urticaria. Br Med J. 1967;4(5574):262–4.

105. Fisher M, Baldo BA. Anaphylaxis during anaesthesia: current aspects of diagnosis and prevention. Eur J Anaesthesiol. 1994;11(4):263–84.

106. Fisher MM, Baldo BA. The incidence and clinical features of anaphylactic reactions during anesthesia in Australia. Ann Fr Anesth Reanim. 1993;12(2):97–104.

107. Mirakian R, Ewan PW, Durham SR, Youlten LJ, Dugue P, Friedmann PS, et al. BSACI guidelines for the management of drug allergy. Clin Exp Allergy. 2009;39(1):43–61.

108. Salvo F, Polimeni G, Cutroneo PM, Leone R, Confortic A, Moretti U, Motola D, Tuccori M, Caputi AP. Allergic reactions to oral drugs: a case/non-case study from an Italian spontaneous reporting database (GIF). Pharmacol Res. 2008;58:202–7.

109. Tang ML, Osborne N, Allen K. Epidemiology of anaphylaxis. Curr Opin Allergy Clin Immunol. 2009;9:351–6.

110. Liew WK, Williamson E, Tang ML. Anaphylaxis fatalities and admissions in Australia. J Allergy Clin Immunol. 2009;123:434–42.

111. Pumphrey RS, Roberts IS. Postmortem findings after fatal anaphylactic reactions. J Clin Pathol. 2000;53:273–6.

112. Low I, Stables S. Anaphylactic deaths in Auckland, New Zealand: a review of coronial autopsies from 1985 to 2005. Pathology. 2006;38:328–32.

113. Brown AF, McKinnon D, Chu K. Emergency department anaphylaxis: a review of 142 patients in a single year. J Allergy Clin Immunol. 2001;108:861–6.

114. Idsoe O, Guthe T, Willcox RR, DeWeck AL. Nature and extent of penicillin side-reactions, with particular reference to fatalities from anaphylactic shock. Bull World Health Organ. 1968;38:159–88.

115. Valentine M, Frank M, Friedland L. Allergic emergencies. In: Drause RM, editor. Asthma and other allergic diseases, NIAID Task Force Report. Bethesda, MD: National Institutes of Health; 1979. p. 467–507.

116. Joint Task Force on Practice Parameters, American Academy of Allergy, Asthma and Immunology, American College of Allergy, Asthma and Immunology, Joint Council of Allergy, Asthma and Immunology. The diagnosis and management of anaphylaxis: an updated practice parameter. J Allergy Clin Immunol. 2005;115(Suppl 2):S483–523.

117. Fisher MM, Baldo BA. The incidence and clinical features of anaphylactic reactions during anesthesia in Australia. Ann Fr Anesth Reanim. 1993;12:97–104.

118. Mertes PM, Laxenaire MC, GERAP. Anaphylactic and anaphylactoid reactions occurring during anaesthesia in France. Seventh epidemiologic survey (January 2001-December 2002). Ann Fr Anesth Reanim. 2004;23:1133–43.

119. Thienthong S, Hintong T, Pulnitiporn A. The Thai Anesthesia Incidents Study (THAI Study) of perioperative allergic reactions. J Med Assoc Thail. 2005;88(Suppl 7):S128–33.

120. Watkins J. Adverse anaesthetic reactions: an update from a proposed national reporting and advisory service. Anaesthesia. 1985;40:797–800.

121. Harboe T, Guttormsen AB, Irgens A, Dybendal T, Florvaag E. Anaphylaxis during anesthesia in Norway: a 6-year single-center follow-up study. Anesthesiology. 2005;102:897–903.

122. Mertes PM, Lambert M, Guéant-Rodriguez RM, Aimone-Gastin I, Mouton-Faivre C, Moneret-Vautrin DA, Guéant JL, Malinovsky JM, Demoly P. Perioperative anaphylaxis. Immunol Allergy Clin N Am. 2009;29:429–51.

123. Schneck J, Fagot JP, Sekula P, Sassolas B, Roujeau JC, Mockenhaupt M. Effects of treatments on the mortality of Stevens-Johnson syndrome and toxic epidermal necrolysis: a retrospective study on patients included in the prospective EuroSCAR Study. J Am Acad Dermatol. 2008;58:33–40.

124. Gamboa PM. The epidemiology of drug allergy-related consultations in Spanish Allergology Services: Alergológica-2005. J Investig Allergol Clin Immunol. 2009;19(Suppl. 2):45–50.

125. Gomes E, Cardoso MF, Praça F, Gomes L, Mariño E, Demoly P. Self-reported drug allergy in a general adult Portuguese population. Clin Exp Allergy. 2004;34:1597–601.

126. Barranco P, Lopez-Serrano MC. General and epidemiological aspects of allergic drug reactions. Clin Exp Allergy. 1998;28(Suppl 4):S61–2.

127. Haddi E, Charpin D, Tafforeau M, Kulling G, Lanteaume A, Kleisbauer JP, Vervloet D. Atopy and systemic reactions to drugs. Allergy. 1990;45:236–9.

128. Leong KP, Thong BY, Cheng YK, Tang CY, Chng HH. Are there differences in drug allergy between the sexes? Ann Acad Med Singap. 2003;32:151.

129. Impicciatore P, Choonara I, Clarkson A, Provasi D, Pandolfini C, Bonati M. Incidence of adverse drug reactions in paediatric in/outpatients: a systematic review and meta-analysis of prospective studies. Br J Clin Pharmacol. 2001;52:77–83.

130. Demoly P, Bousquet J. Epidemiology of drug allergy. Curr Opin Allergy Clin Immunol. 2001;1:305–10.

131. Chng HH, Leong KP, Cheng YK, Tang CY, Chia FL, Tan JW, Thong BY. Elderly inpatients have drug allergy manifestations and outcome similar to the non-elderly but serious reactions are less common: results of a 9-year prospective study. Allergy. 2008;63(Suppl 88):379.

132. Pope J, Jerome D, Fenlon D, Krizova A, Ouimet J. Frequency of adverse drug reactions in patients with systemic lupus erythematosus. J Rheumatol. 2003;30:480–4.

133. Phillips E, Mallal S. Drug hypersensitivity in HIV. Curr Opin Allergy Clin Immunol. 2007;7:324–30.

134. Chung WH, Hung SI, Hong HS, Hsih MS, Yang LC, Ho HC, et al. Medical genetics: a marker for Stevens-Johnson syndrome. Nature. 2004;428:486.

135. McKenna JK, Leiferman KM. Dermatologic drug reactions. Immunol Allergy Clin N Am. 2004;24:399–423.

136. Blanca M, Mayorga C, Torres MJ, et al. Clinical evaluation of Pharmacia CAP System RAST FEIA amoxicilloyl and benzylpenicilloyl in patients with penicillin allergy. Allergy. 2001;56:862–70.

137. Fontaine C, Mayorga C, Bousquet PJ, et al. Relevance of the determination of serum-specific IgE antibodies in the diagnosis of immediate beta-lactam allergy. Allergy. 2007;62:47–52.

138. Sanz ML, Maselli JP, Gamboa PM, et al. Flow cytometric basophil activation test: a review. J Investig Allergol Clin Immunol. 2002;12:143–254.

139. Gamboa P, Sanz ML, Caballero MR, et al. The flow-cytometric determination of basophil activation induced by aspirin and other nonsteroidal anti-inflammatory drugs (NSAIDs) is useful for in vitro diagnosis of the NSAID hypersensitivity syndrome. Clin Exp Allergy. 2004;34:1448–57.

140. Sanz ML, Gamboa PM, Antepara I, et al. Flow cytometric basophil activation test by detection of CD63 expression in patients with immediate-type reactions to betalactam antibiotics. Clin Exp Allergy. 2002;32:277–86.

141. Torres MJ, Padial A, Mayorga C, et al. The diagnostic interpretation of basophil activation test in immediate allergic reactions to betalactams. Clin Exp Allergy. 2004;34:1768–75.

142. Romano A, Viola M, Mondino C, et al. Diagnosing nonimmediatereactions to penicillins by in vivo tests. Int Arch Allergy Immunol. 2002;129:169–74.

143. Barbaud A, Reichert-Penetrat S, Trechot P, et al. The use of skin testing in the investigation of cutaneous adverse drug reactions. Br J Dermatol. 1998;139:49–58.

144. Britschgi M, Steiner UC, Schmid S, et al. T-cell involvement in drug-induced acute generalized exanthematous pustulosis. J Clin Invest. 2001;107:1433–41.

145. Cuerda Galindo E, Goday Bujan JJ, Garcia Silva JM, et al. Fixed drug eruption from piroxicam. J Eur Acad Dermatol Venereol. 2004;18:586–7.

146. Wolkenstein P, Chosidow O, Flechet ML, et al. Patch testing in severe cutaneous adverse drug reactions, including Stevens-Johnson syndrome and toxic epidermal necrolysis. Contact Dermatitis. 1996;35:234–6.

147. Bronnimann M, Yawalkar N. Histopathology of drug-induced exanthems: is there a role in diagnosis of drug allergy? Curr Opin Allergy Clin Immunol. 2005;5:317–21.

148. Sogn DD, Evans R, Shepherd GM, et al. Results of the National Institute of Allergy and Infectious Diseases collaborative clinical trial to test the predictive value of skin testing with major and

minor penicillin derivatives in hospitalized adults. Ann Intern Med. 1992;152:1025–32.

149. Gadde J, Spence M, Wheeler B, et al. Clinical experience with penicillin skin testing in a large inner-city STD clinic. JAMA. 1993;270:2456–63.

150. Lee CE, Zembower TR, Fotis MA, et al. The incidence of antimicrobial allergies in hospitalized patients: implications regarding prescribing patterns and emerging bacterial resistance. Ann Intern Med. 2000;160:2819–22.

151. Green GR, Rosenblum AH. Report of the penicillin study group, American Academy of Allergy. J Allergy Clin Immunol. 1971;48:331–43.

152. del Real GA, Rose ME, Ramirez-Atamoros MT, et al. Penicillin skin testing in patients with a history of beta-lactam allergy. Ann Allergy Asthma Immunol. 2007;98:355–9.

153. Romano A, Gueant-Rodriguez RM, Viola M, et al. Cross-reactivity and tolerability of cephalosporins in patients with immediate hypersensitivity to penicillins. Ann Intern Med. 2004;141:16–22.

154. Pumphrey RSH, Davis S. Under-reporting of antibiotic anaphylaxis may put patients at risk. Lancet. 1999;353:1157–8.

155. Park M, Markus P, Matesic D, et al. Safety and effectiveness of a preoperative allergy clinic in decreasing vancomycin use in patients with a history of penicillin allergy. Ann Allergy Asthma Immunol. 2006;97:681–7.

156. Romano A, Viola M, Gueant-Rodriguez RM, et al. Tolerability of meropenem in patients with IgE-mediated hypersensitivity to penicillins. Ann Intern Med. 2007;146:266–9.

157. Romano A, Viola M, Gueant-Rodriquez RA, et al. Imipenem in patients with immediate hypersensitivity to penicillins. N Engl J Med. 2006;354:2835–7.

158. Baur X, Bossert J, Koops F. IgE-mediated allergy to recombinant human insulin in a diabetic. Allergy. 2003;58:676–8.

159. Heinzerling L, Raile K, Rochlitz H, et al. Insulin allergy: clinical manifestations and management strategies. Allergy. 2008;63:148–55.

160. Nagai Y, Mori T, Abe T, et al. Immediate-type allergy against human insulin associated with marked eosinophilia in type 2 diabetic patient. Endocr J. 2001;48:311–6.

161. Schernthaner G. Immunogenicity and allergenic potential of animal and human insulins. Diabetes Care. 1993;16(suppl 3):155–65.

162. Adachi A, Fukunaga A, Horikawa T. A case of human insulin allergy induced by short-acting and intermediate-acting insulin but not by long-acting insulin. Int J Dermatol. 2004;43:597–9.

163. Castera V, Dutour-Meyer A, Koeppel M, et al. Systemic allergy to human insulin and its rapid and long acting analogs: successful treatment by continuous subcutaneous insulin lispro infusion. Diabetes Metab. 2005;31(4 pt 1):391–400.

164. Brange J, Andersen L, Laursen ED, et al. Toward understanding insulin fibrillation. J Pharm Sci. 1997;86:517–25.

165. Eisenhauer EA, ten Bokkel-Huinink WW, Swenerton KD, et al. European-Canadian randomized trial of paclitaxel in relapsed ovarian cancer: high-dose versus low-dose and long versus short infusion. J Clin Oncol. 1994;12:2654–66.

166. Markman M, Kennedy A, Webster K, et al. Paclitaxel-associated hypersensitivity reactions: experience of the gynecologic oncology program of the Cleveland Clinic Cancer Center. J Clin Oncol. 2000;18:102–5.

167. Lee CW, Matulonis UA, Castells MC. Carboplatin hypersensitivity: a 12-step protocol effective in 35 desensitizations in patients with gynecological malignancies and mast cell/IgE-mediated reactions. Gynecol Oncol. 2004;95:370–6.

168. Essayan DM, Kagey-Sobotka A, Colarusso PJ, et al. Successful parental desensitization to paclitaxel. J Allergy Clin Immunol. 1996;97:42–6.

169. Castells MC, Tennant NM, Sloane DE, et al. Hypersensitivity reactions to chemotherapy: outcomes and safety of rapid desensitization in 413 cases. J Allergy Clin Immunol. 2008;122:574–80.

170. Bernstein BJ. Docetaxel as an alternative to paclitaxel after acute hypersensitivity reactions. Ann Pharmacother. 2000;11:1332–5.

171. Polyzos A, Tsavaris N, Kosmas C, et al. Hypersensitivity reactions to carboplatin administration are common but not always severe: a 10-year experience. Oncology. 2001;61:129–33.

172. Zanotti KM, Rybicki LA, Kennedy AW, et al. Carboplatin skin testing: a skin-testing protocol for predicting hypersensitivity to carboplatin chemotherapy. J Clin Oncol. 2001;19:3126–9.

173. Goldberg A, Confino-Cohen R, Fishman A, et al. A modified, prolonged desensitization protocol in carboplatin allergy. J Allergy Clin Immunol. 1996;98:841–3.

174. Markman M, Zanotti K, Peterson G, et al. Expanded experience with an intradermal skin test to predict for the presence or absence of carboplatin hypersensitivity. J Clin Oncol. 2003;21:4611–4.

175. Garufi C, Cristaudo A, Vanni B, et al. Skin testing and hypersensitivity reactions to oxaliplatin. Ann Oncol. 2003;14:497–8.

176. Lee BL, Safrin S. Interactions and toxicities of drugs used in patients with AIDS. Clin Infect Dis. 1992;14:773–9.

177. Koopmans PP, vanderVen AJ, Vree TB, et al. Pathogenesis of hypersensitivity reactions to drugs in patients with HIV infection: allergic or toxic? AIDS. 1995;9:217–22.
178. Carr A, Cooper DA, Penny R. Allergic manifestations of human immunodeficiency virus (HIV) infection. J Clin Immunol. 1991;11:55–64.
179. Carr A, Swanson R, Penny R, et al. Clinical and laboratory markers of hypersensitivity to trimethoprim-sulphamethoxazole in patients with Pneumocystis carinii pneumonia and AIDS. J Infect Dis. 1993;167:180–5.
180. Bayard P, Berger T, Jacobson M. Drug hypersensitivity reactions and human immunodeficiency virus disease. J Acquir Immune Defic Syndr. 1992;5:1237–57.
181. Absar N, Daneshvar H, Beall G. Desensitization to trimethoprim/sulfamethoxazole in HIV-infected patients. J Allergy Clin Immunol. 1994;93:1001–5.
182. Gluckstein D, Ruskin J. Rapid oral desensitization to trimethoprimsulfathoxazole (TMP-SMZ): use in prophylaxis for Pneumocystis carini pneumonia in patients with AIDS who were previously intolerant to TMP-SMZ. Clin Infect Dis. 1995;20:849–53.
183. Nguyen M, Weiss PJ, Wallace MR. Two-day oral desensitization to trimethoprim-sulfamethoxazole in HIV-infected patients. AIDS. 1995;9:573–5.
184. Belchi-Hernandez J, Espinosa-Parra FJ. Management of adverse reactions to prophylactic trimethoprim-sulfamethoxazole in patients with human immunodeficiency virus infection. Ann Allergy Asthma Immunol. 1996;76:355–8.
185. Kalanadhabhatta V, Muppidi D, Sahni H, et al. Successful oral desensitization to trimethoprim-sulfamethoxazole in acquired immune deficiency syndrome. Ann Allergy Asthma Immunol. 1996;77:394–400.
186. Caumes E, Guermonprez G, Lecomte C, et al. Efficacy and safety of desensitization with sulfamethoxazole and trimethoprim in 48 previously hypersensitive patients infected with human immunodeficiency virus. Arch Dermatol. 1997;133:465–9.
187. Rich JD, Sullivan T, Greineder D, et al. Trimethoprim/sulfamethoxazole incremental dose regimen in human immunodeficiency virus-infected persons. Ann Allergy Asthma Immunol. 1997;79:409–14.
188. Ryan C, Madalon M, Wortham DW, et al. Sulfa hypersensitivity in patients with HIV infection: onset, treatment, critical review of the literature. Wis Med J. 1998;97:23–7.

189. Demoly P, Messaad D, Sahla H, et al. Six-hour trimethoprim sulfamethoxazole-graded challenge in HIV-infected patients. J Allergy Clin Immunol. 1998;102(6 pt 1):1033–6.

190. Bonfanti P, Pusterla L, Parazzini F, et al. The effectiveness of desensitization versus rechallenge treatment in HIV-positive patients with previous hypersensitivity to TMP-SMX: a randomized multicentric study. Biomed Pharmacother. 2000;54:45–9.

191. Yoshizawa S, Yasuoka A, Kikuchi Y, et al. A 5-day course of oral desensitization to trimethoprim/sulfamethoxazole (T/S) in patients with human immunodeficiency virus type-1 infection who were previously intolerant to T/S. Ann Allergy Asthma Immunol. 2000;85:241–4.

192. Moreno JN, Poblete RB, Maggio C, et al. Rapid oral desensitization for sulfonamides in patients with the acquired immunodeficiency syndrome. Ann Allergy Asthma Immunol. 1995;74:140–6.

193. Tenant-Flowers M, Boyle MJ, Carey D, et al. Sulphadiazine desensitization in patients with AIDS and cerebral toxoplasmosis. AIDS. 1991;5:311–5.

194. Carr A, Penny R, Cooper DA. Allergy and desensitization to zidovudine in patients with acquired immunodeficiency syndrome (AIDS). J Allergy Clin Immunol. 1993;91:683–5.

195. Henry RE, Wegmann JA, Hartle JE, et al. Successful oral acyclovir desensitization. Ann Allergy. 1993;70:386–8.

196. Duque S, delaPuente J, Rodriguez F, et al. Zidovudine-related erythroderma and successful desensitization: a case report. J Allergy Clin Immunol. 1996;98:234–5.

197. Cook DE, Kossey JL. Successful desensitization to dapsone for Pneumocystis carinii prophylaxis in an HIV-positive patient. Ann Pharmacother. 1998;32:1302–5.

198. Metroka CE, Lewis NJ, Jacobus DP. Desensitization to dapsone in HIV-positive patients [letter]. JAMA. 1992;267:512.

199. McNeill O, Kerridge RK, Boyle MJ. Review of procedures for investigation of anaesthesia-associated anaphylaxis in Newcastle, Australia. Anaesth Intensive Care. 2008;36:201–7.

200. Weiss ME, Nyhan D, Peng ZK, et al. Association of protamine IgE and IgG antibodies with life-threatening reactions to intravenous protamine. N Engl J Med. 1989;320:886–92.

201. Vincent GM, Janowski M, Menlove R. Protamine allergy reactions during cardiac catheterization and cardiac surgery: risk in patients taking protamine-insulin preparations. Cathet Cardiovasc Diagn. 1991;23:164–8.

202. Gottschlich GM, Gravlee GP, Georgitis JW. Adverse reactions to protamine sulfate during cardiac surgery in diabetic and non-diabetic patients. Ann Allergy. 1988;61:277–81.

203. Stewart WJ, McSweeney SM, Kellett MA, et al. Increased risk of severe protamine reactions in NPH insulin-dependent diabetics undergoing cardiac catheterization. Circulation. 1984;70:788–92.
204. Cherry T, Steciuk M, Reddy VV, et al. Transfusion-related acute lung injury: past, present, and future. Am J Clin Pathol. 2008;129:287–97.
205. Goldman M, Webert KE, Arnold DM, et al. Proceedings of a consensus conference: towards an understanding of TRALI. Transfus Med Rev. 2005;19:2–31.
206. Peller JS, Bardana EJ. Anaphylactoid reaction to corticosteroid: case report and review of the literature. Ann Allergy. 1986;54:302–5.
207. Freedman MD, Schocket AL, Chapel N, et al. Anaphylaxis after intravenous methylprednisolone administration. JAMA. 1981;245:607–8.
208. Mendelson LM, Meltzer EO, Hamburger RN. Anaphylaxis-like reactions to corticosteroid therapy. J Allergy Clin Immunol. 1974;54:125–31.
209. Butani L. Corticosteroid-induced hypersensitivity reactions. Ann Allergy Asthma Immunol. 2002;89:439–45.
210. Burgdorff T, Venemalm L, Vogt T, et al. IgE-medicated anaphylactic reaction induced by succinate ester of methylprednisolone. Ann Allergy Asthma Immunol. 2002;89:425–8.
211. Rasanen L, Tarvainen K, Makinen-Kiljunen S. Urticaria to hydrocortisone. Allergy. 2001;56:352–3.
212. Warkentin TE, Greinacher A. Heparin-induced thrombocytopenia: recognition, treatment, and prevention: the Seventh ACCP Conference on Antithrombotic and Thrombolytic Therapy. Chest. 2004;126:311S–37S.
213. Kishimoto TK, Viswanathan K, Ganguly T, et al. Contaminated heparin associated with adverse clinical events and activation of the contact system. N Engl J Med. 2008;358:2457–67.
214. Cuesta-Herranz J, de las Heras M, Fernandez M, et al. Allergic reaction caused by local anesthetic agents belonging to the amide group. J Allergy Clin Immunol. 1997;99:427–8.
215. Gonzalez-Delgado P, Anton R, Soriano V, et al. Cross-reactivity among amide-type local anesthetics in a case of allergy to mepivacaine. J Investig Allergol Clin Immunol. 2006;16:311–3.
216. Prieto A, Herrero T, Rubio M, et al. Urticaria due to mepivacaine with tolerance to lidocaine and bupivacaine. Allergy. 2005;60:261–2.
217. Venemalm L, Degerbeck F, Smith W. IgE-mediated reaction to mepivacaine. J Allergy Clin Immunol. 2008;121:1058–9.

218. Coleman WP, Ochsner SF, Watson BE. Allergic reactions in 10,000 consecutive intravenous urographies. South Med. 1964;57:1401–4.

219. Wolf GL, Mishkin MM, Roux SG, et al. Comparison of the rates of adverse drug reactions: ionic contrast agents, ionic agents combined with steroids, and nonionic agents. Investig Radiol. 1991;26:404–10.

220. Katayama H, Yamaguchi K, Kozuka T, et al. Adverse reactions to ionic and nonionic contrast media: a report from the Japanese Committee on the Safety of Contrast Media. Radiology. 1990;175:621–8.

221. Lang DM, Alpern MB, Visintainer PF, et al. Gender risk for anaphylactoid reaction to radiographic contrast media. J Allergy Clin Immunol. 1995;95:813–7.

222. Enricht T, Chau-Lim E, Duda E, et al. The role of a documented allergic profile as a risk factor for radiographic contrast media reaction. Ann Allergy. 1989;62:302–5.

223. Schatz M, Patterson R, O'Rourke J, et al. The administration of radiographic contrast media to patients with a history of a previous reaction. J Allergy Clin Immunol. 1975;55:358–66.

224. Lang DM, Alpern MB, Visintainer PF, et al. Increased risk for anaphylactoid reaction from contrast media in patients on beta-adrenergic blockers or with asthma. Ann Intern Med. 1991;115:270–6.

225. Lang DM, Alpern MB, Visintainer PF, et al. Elevated risk of anaphylactoid reaction from radiographic contrast media is associated with both beta-blocker exposure and cardiovascular disorders. Ann Intern Med. 1993;153:2033–40.

226. Arm JP, O'Hickey SP, Hawksworth RJ, et al. Asthmatic airways have a disproportionate hyperresponsiveness to LTE4, as compared with normal airways, but not to LTC4, LTD4, methacholine, and histamine. Am Rev Respir Dis. 1990;142:1112–8.

227. Sousa AR, Parikh A, Scadding G, et al. Leukotriene-receptor expression on nasal mucosal inflammatory cells in aspirin-sensitive rhinosinusitis. N Engl J Med. 2002;347:1493–9. IIa.

228. Martin-Garcia C, Hinojosa M, Berges P, et al. Safety of a cyclooxygenase-2 inhibitor in patients with aspirin-sensitive asthma. Chest. 2002;121:1812–7.

229. Gyllfors P, Bochenek G, Overholt J, et al. Biochemical and clinical evidence that aspirin-intolerant asthmatic subjects tolerate the cyclooxygenase 2-selective analgetic drug celecoxib. J Allergy Clin Immunol. 2003;111:1116–21.

230. Woessner K, Simon RA, Stevenson DD. The safety of celecoxib in aspirin exacerbated respiratory disease. Arthritis Rheum. 2002;46:2201–6.

231. Stevenson DD, Simon RA. Lack of cross-reactivity between rofecoxib and aspirin in aspirin-sensitive patients with asthma. J Allergy Clin Immunol. 2001;108:47–51.
232. Baldassarre S, Schandene L, Choufani G, et al. Asthma attacks induced by low doses of celecoxib, aspirin, and acetaminophen. J Allergy Clin Immunol. 2006;117:215–7.
233. Tracy JM. Insect allergy. Mt Sinai J Med. 2011;78(5):773–83. https://doi.org/10.1002/msj.20286.
234. Burns BD. Insect bites medication. In: Alcock J, editor. Medscape. http://emedicine.medscape.com/article/769067-medication#showall. Accessed 27 June 2016.
235. Krishna MT, Ewan PW, Diwakar L, Durham SR, Frew AJ, Leech SC. Diagnosis and management of hymenoptera venom allergy: British Society for Allergy and Clinical Immunology (BSACI) guidelines. Clin Exp Allergy. 2011;41(9):1201–20.
236. Zirngibl G, Burrows HL. Hymenoptera stings. Pediatr Rev. 2012;33(11):534–5; discussion 535.
237. Ewan PW. Venom allergy. BMJ. 1998;316(7141):1365–8.
238. Ewan PW. ABC of allergies. BMJ. 1998;316:1442–5.
239. Golden DB. Insect sting anaphylaxis. Immunol Allergy Clin N Am. 2007;27(2):261–72.
240. Hoffman DR, Jacobson RS, Schmidt M, Smith AM. Allergens in Hymenoptera venoms. XXIII. Venom content of imported fire ant whole body extracts. Ann Allergy. 1991;66:29–31.
241. Golden DB. Anaphylaxis to insect stings. Immunol Allergy Clin N Am. 2015;35(2):287–302. https://doi.org/10.1016/j.iac.2015.01.007.
242. Novembre E, Cianferoni A, Bernardini RA, Ingargiola A, Lombardi E, Vierucci A. Epidemiology of insect venom sensitivity in children and its correlation to clinical and atopic features. Clin Exp Allergy. 1998;28:834–8.
243. Dhami S, Nurmatov U, Varga EM, Sturm G, Muraro A, Akdis CA, Antolín-Amérigo D, et al. Allergen immunotherapy for insect venom allergy: protocol for a systematic review. Clin Trans Allergy. 2016;6:6. https://doi.org/10.1186/s13601-016-0095-x; eCollection 2015.
244. Mowry JB, Spyker DA, Brooks DE, McMillan N, Schauben JL. 2014 Annual Report of the American Association of Poison Control Centers' National Poison Data System (NPDS): 32nd Annual Report. Clin Toxicol (Phila). 2015;53(10):962–1147.
245. Golden DBK, Marsh DG, Kagey-Sobotka A, Addison BI, Freidhoff L, Szklo M, et al. Epidemiology of insect venom sensitivity. JAMA. 1989;262:240–4.
246. Settipane GA, Newstead GJ, Boyd GK. Frequency of Hymenoptera allergy in an atopic and normal population. J Allergy. 1972;50:146–50.

247. Barnard JH. Studies of 400 hymenoptera sting deaths in the United States. J Allergy Clin Immunol. 1973;52:259–64.
248. Hoffman DR. Fatal reactions to hymenoptera stings. Allergy Asthma Proc. 2003;24:123–7.
249. Schwartz HJ, Sutheimer C, Gauerke B, Zora JA, Yunginger JW. Venom-specific IgE antibodies in postmortem sera from victims of sudden unexpected death. J Allergy Clin Immunol. 1984;73:189.
250. Golden DBK, Marsh DG, Freidhoff LR, Kwiterovich KA, Addison B, Kagey-Sobotka A, et al. Natural history of Hymenoptera venom sensitivity in adults. J Allergy Clin Immunol. 1997;100:760–6.
251. Clark S, Camargo CA Jr. Epidemiology of anaphylaxis. Immunol Allergy Clin N Am. 2007;27(2):145–63.
252. Pumphrey RSH. Lessons for management of anaphylaxis from a study of fatal reactions. Clin Exp Allergy. 2000;30(8):1144–50.
253. Krishna MT, Ewan PM, Diwakar L, Durham SR, Frew AJ, Leech SC, Nasser SM. Diagnosis and management of hymenoptera venom allergy: British Society for Allergy and Clinical Immunology (BSACI) guidelines. Clin Exp Allergy. 2011;41:1201–20.
254. Stritzke AI, Eng PA. Age-dependent sting recurrence and outcome in immunotherapy-treated children with anaphylaxis to hymenoptera venom. Clin Exp Allergy. 2013;43(8):950–5.
255. Bilò BM, Bonifazi F. Epidemiology of insect-venom anaphylaxis. Curr Opin Allergy Clin Immunol. 2008;8(4):330–7.
256. Aalberse RC, Koshte V, Clemens JGJ. Immunoglobulin E antibodies that crossreact with vegetable foods, pollen, and Hymenoptera venom. J Allergy Clin Immunol. 1981;68:356–64.
257. Hemmer W, Frocke M, Kolarich K, Wilson IBH, Altmann F, Wohrl S, et al. Antibody binding to venom carbohydrates is a frequent cause for double positivity to honeybee and yellow jacket venom in patients with stinging insect allergy. J Allergy Clin Immunol. 2001;108:1045–52.
258. Hamilton RG. Diagnostic methods for insect sting allergy. Curr Opin Allergy Clin Immunol. 2004;4:297–306.
259. Goldberg A, Confino-Cohen R. Timing of venom skin tests and IgE determinations after insect sting anaphylaxis. J Allergy Clin Immunol. 1997;100:183–4.
260. Centers for Disease Control and Prevention. Insects and scorpions. http://www.cdc.gov/niosh/topics/insects. Accessed 31 July 2014.
261. Simons FE, Ardusso LR, Bilò MB, et al. 2012 update: World Allergy Organization guidelines for the assessment and management of anaphylaxis. Curr Opin Allergy Clin Immunol. 2012;12(4):389–99.

262. Erbilen E, Gulcan E, Albayrak S, Ozveren O. Acute myocardial infarction due to a bee sting manifested with ST wave elevation after hospital admission. South Med J. 2008;101(4):448.

263. Moffitt JE, Golden DBK, Reisman RE, Lee R, Nicklas R, Freeman T, et al. Stinging insect hypersensitivity: a practice parameter update. J Allergy Clin Immunol. 2004;114:869–86.

264. Golden DBK, Kwiterovich KA, Kagey-Sobotka A, Valentine MD, Lichtenstein LM. Discontinuing venom immunotherapy: outcome after five years. J Allergy Clin Immunol. 1996;97:579–87.

265. Golden DBK, Kwiterovich KA, Addison BA, Kagey-Sobotka A, Lichtenstein LM. Discontinuing venom immunotherapy: extended observations. J Allergy Clin Immunol. 1998;101:298–305.

266. Allergy. http://www.birmingham.ac.uk/Documents/college-mds/facilities/cis/Essentialimmunology/Chapter3.pdf. Accessed 30 June 2016.

267. Busse WW, Calhoun WF, Sedgwick JD. Mechanism of airway inflammation in asthma. Am Rev Respir Dis. 1993;147(6 Pt 2):S20–4.

268. Horwitz RJ, Busse WW. Inflammation and asthma. Clin Chest Med. 1995;16(4):583–602.

269. Morris MJ. Asthma. In: Mosenifar Z, editor. Medscape. http://emedicine.medscape.com/article/296301-overview#a2. Accessed 30 June 2016.

270. Balzar S, Fajt ML, Comhair SA, Erzurum SC, Bleecker E, Busse WW, et al. Mast cell phenotype, location, and activation in severe asthma: data from the severe asthma research program. Am J Respir Crit Care Med. 2011;183(3):299–309.

271. Gauvreau GM, Boulet LP, Cockcroft DW, et al. Effects of interleukin-13 blockade on allergen-induced airway responses in mild atopic asthma. Am J Respir Crit Care Med. 2011;183(8):1007–14.

272. Anderson WJ, Watson L. Asthma and the hygiene hypothesis. N Engl J Med. 2001;344(21):1643–4.

273. Brooks C, Pearce N, Douwes J. The hygiene hypothesis in allergy and asthma: an update. Curr Opin Allergy Clin Immunol. 2013;13(1):70–7.

274. Sears MR. Consequences of long-term inflammation. The natural history of asthma. Clin Chest Med. 2000;21(2):315–29.

275. Camargo CA Jr, Weiss ST, Zhang S, Willett WC, Speizer FE. Prospective study of body mass index, weight change, and risk of adult-onset asthma in women. Arch Intern Med. 1999;159(21):2582–8.

276. Emergency Asthma Treatment. WebMD. http://www.webmd.com/asthma/asthma-emergency-treatment. Accessed 30 June 2016.

277. Iribarren C, Tolstykh IV, Miller MK, Eisner MD. Asthma and the prospective risk of anaphylactic shock and other allergy diagnoses in a large integrated health care delivery system.

Ann Allergy Asthma Immunol. 2010;104(5):371–7. https://doi.org/10.1016/j.anai.2010.03.004.

278. González-Pérez A, Aponte Z, Vidaurre CF, Rodríguez LA. Anaphylaxis epidemiology in patients with and patients without asthma: a United Kingdom database review. J Allergy Clin Immunol. 2010;125(5):1098–1104.e1. https://doi.org/10.1016/j.jaci.2010.02.009; Epub 2010 Apr 14.

279. Sheikh J. Allergic rhinitis. In: Kaliner MA, editor. Medscape. http://emedicine.medscape.com/article/134825-overview. Accessed 30 June 2016.

280. Skoner DP. Allergic rhinitis: definition, epidemiology, pathophysiology, detection, and diagnosis. J Allergy Clin Immunol. 2001;108(1 Suppl):S2–8.

281. Walls AF, He S, Buckley MG, McEuen AR. Roles of the mast cell and basophil in asthma. Clin Exp Allergy. 2001;1:68.

282. Haberal I, Corey JP. The role of leukotrienes in nasal allergy. Otolaryngol Head Neck Surg. 2003;129(3):274–9.

283. Iwasaki M, Saito K, Takemura M, Sekikawa K, Fujii H, Yamada Y. TNF-alpha contributes to the development of allergic rhinitis in mice. J Allergy Clin Immunol. 2003;112(1):134–40.

284. Cates EC, Gajewska BU, Goncharova S, Alvarez D, Fattouh R, Coyle AJ. Effect of GM-CSF on immune, inflammatory, and clinical responses to ragweed in a novel mouse model of mucosal sensitization. J Allergy Clin Immunol. 2003;111(5):1076–86.

285. Salib RJ, Kumar S, Wilson SJ, Howarth PH. Nasal mucosal immunoexpression of the mast cell chemoattractants TGF-beta, eotaxin, and stem cell factor and their receptors in allergic rhinitis. J Allergy Clin Immunol. 2004;114(4):799–806.

286. Hansen I, Klimek L, Mosges R, Hormann K. Mediators of inflammation in the early and the late phase of allergic rhinitis. Curr Opin Allergy Clin Immunol. 2004;4(3):159–63.

287. Dykewicz MS, Fineman S, Skoner DP, Nicklas R, Lee R, Blessing-Moore J. Diagnosis and management of rhinitis: complete guidelines of the Joint Task Force on Practice Parameters in Allergy, Asthma and Immunology. American Academy of Allergy, Asthma, and Immunology. Ann Allergy Asthma Immunol. 1998;81(5 Pt 2):478–518.

288. Frew AJ. Advances in environmental and occupational diseases 2003. J Allergy Clin Immunol. 2004;113(6):1161–6.

289. Boulet LP, Turcotte H, Laprise C, Lavertu C, Bedard PM, Lavoie A. Comparative degree and type of sensitization to common indoor and outdoor allergens in subjects with allergic rhinitis and/or asthma. Clin Exp Allergy. 1997;27(1):52–9.

290. Watson WT, Becker AB, Simons FE. Treatment of allergic rhinitis with intranasal corticosteroids in patients with mild asthma:

effect on lower airway responsiveness. J Allergy Clin Immunol. 1993;91(1 Pt 1):97–101.

291. Meltzer EO, Grant JA. Impact of cetirizine on the burden of allergic rhinitis. Ann Allergy Asthma Immunol. 1999;83(5):455–63.

292. Kiyohara C, Tanaka K, Miyake Y. Genetic susceptibility to atopic dermatitis. Allergol Int. 2008;57(1):39–56.

293. Nayak AS. The asthma and allergic rhinitis link. Allergy Asthma Proc. 2003;24(6):395–402.

294. Colás C, Galera H, Añibarro B, Soler R, Navarro A, Jáuregui I, et al. Disease severity impairs sleep quality in allergic rhinitis (The SOMNIAAR study). Clin Exp Allergy. 2012;42(7): 1080–7.

295. Tsai JD, Chang SN, Mou CH, Sung FC, Lue KH. Association between atopic diseases and attention-deficit/hyperactivity disorder in childhood: a population-based case-control study. Ann Epidemiol. 2013;23(4):185–8.

296. Fireman P. Otitis media and eustachian tube dysfunction: connection to allergic rhinitis. J Allergy Clin Immunol. 1997;99(2):S787–97.

297. McColley SA, Carroll JL, Curtis S, Loughlin GM, Sampson HA. High prevalence of allergic sensitization in children with habitual snoring and obstructive sleep apnea. Chest. 1997;111(1):170–3.

298. Craig TJ, Teets S, Lehman EB, Chinchilli VM, Zwillich C. Nasal congestion secondary to allergic rhinitis as a cause of sleep disturbance and daytime fatigue and the response to topical nasal corticosteroids. J Allergy Clin Immunol. 1998;101(5):633–7.

299. Ray NF, Baraniuk JN, Thamer M, Rinehart CS, Gergen PJ, Kaliner M. Direct expenditures for the treatment of allergic rhinoconjunctivitis in 1996, including the contributions of related airway illnesses. J Allergy Clin Immunol. 1999;103(3 Pt 1):401–7.

300. Schnyder B, Pichler WJ. Mechanisms of drug-induced allergy. Mayo Clin Proc. 2009;84(3):268–72. http://www.ncbi.nlm.nih.gov/pmc/articles/PMC2664605/. Accessed 30 June 2016.

301. Chung CH, Mirakhur B, Chan E, et al. Cetuximab-induced anaphylaxis and IgE specific for galactose-α-1,3-galactose. N Engl J Med. 2008;358(11):1109–17.

302. Harboe T, Johansson SG, Florvaag E, Oman H. Pholcodine exposure raises serum IgE in patients with previous anaphylaxis to neuromuscular blocking agents. Allergy. 2007;62(12):1445–50.

303. Kvedariene V, Martins P, Rouanet L, Demoly P. Diagnosis of iodinated contrast media hypersensitivity: results of a 6-year period. Clin Exp Allergy. 2006;36(8):1072–7.

304. Riley RJ, Leeder JS. In vitro analysis of metabolic predisposition to drug hypersensitivity reactions. Clin Exp Immunol. 1995;99(1):1–6.

305. Büdinger L, Hertl M. Immunologic mechanisms in hypersensitivity reactions to metal ions: an overview. Allergy. 2000;55(2):108–15.

306. Naisbitt DJ, Gordon SF, Pirmohamed M, Park BK. Immunological principles of adverse drug reactions: the initiation and propagation of immune responses elicited by drug treatment. Drug Saf. 2000;23(6):483–507.

307. Mora JR, von Andrian HU. T-cell homing specificity and plasticity: new concepts and futures challenges. Trends Immunol. 2006;27(5):235–43; Epub 2006 Mar 31.

308. Ebert LM, Schaerli P, Moser B. Chemokine-mediated control of T cell traffic in lymphoid and peripheral tissues. Mol Immunol. 2005;42(7):799–809; Epub 2004 Nov 23.

309. Birnbaum J, Vervloet D. Allergy to muscle relaxants. Clin Rev Allergy. 1991;9(3–4):281–93.

310. Aster RH. Drug-induced immune cytopenias. Toxicology. 2005;209(2):149–53.

311. Warkentin TE. Drug-induced immune-mediated thrombocytopenia—from purpura to thrombosis. N Engl J Med. 2007;356(9):891–3.

312. Panesar SS, Javad S, de Silva D, Nwaru BI, Hickstein L, Muraro A, et al. The epidemiology of anaphylaxis in Europe: a systematic review. Allergy. 2013;68:1353–61.

313. Cetinkaya F, Incioglu A, Birinci S, Karaman BE, Dokucu AI, Sheikh A. Hospital admissions for anaphylaxis in Istanbul, Turkey. Allergy. 2013;68:128–30.

314. Harduar-Morano L, Simon MR, Watkins S, Blackmore C. A population-based epidemiologic study of emergency department visits for anaphylaxis in Florida. J Allergy Clin Immunol. 2011;128:594–6001.

315. Tupper J, Visser S. Anaphylaxis: a review and update. Can Fam Physician. 2010;56:1009–11.

316. Neugut AI, Ghatak AT, Miller RL. Anaphylaxis in the United States: an investigation into its epidemiology. Arch Intern Med. 2001;161:15–21.

317. Leone R, Conforti A, Venegoni M, Motola D, Moretti U, Meneghelli I, et al. Drug-induced anaphylaxis: case/non-case study based on an Italian pharmacovigilance database. Drug Saf. 2005;28:547–56.

318. Renaudin JM, Beaudouin E, Ponvert C, Demoly P, Moneret-Vautrin DA. Severe drug-induced anaphylaxis: analysis of 333

cases recorded by the Allergy Vigilance Network from 2002 to 2010. Allergy. 2013;68:929–37.

319. Patel TK, Patel PB, Barvaliya MJ, Tripathi CB. Drug-induced anaphylactic reactions in Indian population: a systematic review. Indian J Crit Care Med. 2014;18(12):796–806.

320. Ribeiro-Vaz I, Marques J, Demoly P, Polónia J, Gomes ER. Drug-induced anaphylaxis: a decade review of reporting to the Portuguese Pharmacovigilance Authority. Eur J Clin Pharmacol. 2013;69:673–81.

321. van der Klauw MM, Stricker BH, Herings RM, Cost WS, Valkenburg HA, Wilson JH. A population based case-cohort study of drug-induced anaphylaxis. Br J Clin Pharmacol. 1993;35:400–8.

322. de Silva IL, Mehr SS, Tey D, Tang ML. Paediatric anaphylaxis: a 5 year retrospective review. Allergy. 2008;63:1071–6.

323. Mertes PM, Laxenaire MC, Alla F. Groupe d'Etudes des Réactions Anaphylactoïdes Peranesthésiques. Anaphylactic and anaphylactoid reactions occurring during anesthesia in France in 1999-2000. Anesthesiology. 2003;99:536–45.

324. Lenler-Petersen P, Hansen D, Andersen M, Sørensen HT, Bille H. Drug-related fatal anaphylactic shock in Denmark 1968-1990. A study based on notifications to the Committee on Adverse Drug Reactions. J Clin Epidemiol. 1995;48:1185–8.

325. International Collaborative Study of Severe Anaphylaxis. Risk of anaphylaxis in a hospital population in relation to the use of various drugs: an international study. Pharmacoepidemiol Drug Saf. 2003;12:195–202.

326. Moro MM, Tejedor Alonso MA, Esteban Hernández J, Múgica García MV, Rosado Ingelmo A, Vila Albelda C. Incidence of anaphylaxis and subtypes of anaphylaxis in a general hospital emergency department. J Investig Allergol Clin Immunol. 2011;21:142–9.

327. van Puijenbroek EP, Egberts AC, Meyboom RH, Leufkens HG. Different risks for NSAID-induced anaphylaxis. Ann Pharmacother. 2002;36:24–9.

328. Laxenaire MC, Mertes PM. Groupe d'Etudes des Réactions Anaphylactoïdes Peranesthésiques. Anaphylaxis during anaesthesia. Results of a two-year survey in France. Br J Anaesth. 2001;87:549–58.

329. Sadleir PH, Clarke RC, Bunning DL, Platt PR. Anaphylaxis to neuromuscular blocking drugs: incidence and cross-reactivity in Western Australia from 2002 to 2011. Br J Anaesth. 2013;110:981–7.

330. Riedl MA, Casillas AM. Adverse drug reactions: types and treatment options. Am Fam Physician. 2003;68(9):1781–91.

331. Saxon A, Adelman DC, Patel A, Hajdu R, Calandra GB. Imipenem cross-reactivity with penicillin in humans. J Allergy Clin Immunol. 1988;82:213–7.

332. Saxon A, Hassner A, Swabb EA, Wheeler B, Adkinson NFJR. Lack of cross-reactivity between aztreonam, a monobactam antibiotic, and penicillin in penicillin-allergic subjects. J Infect Dis. 1984;149:16–22.

333. Adkinson NF Jr. Immunogenicity and cross-allergenicity of aztreonam. Am J Med. 1990;88:12S–5S.

334. Shepherd GM. Allergy to betalactam antibiotics. Immunol Allergy Clin N Am. 1991;11:611–33.

335. Lin RY. A perspective on penicillin allergy. Arch Intern Med. 1992;152:930–7.

336. Kelkar PS, Li JT. Cephalosporin allergy. N Engl J Med. 2001;345:804–9.

337. Executive summary of disease management of drug hypersensitivity: a practice parameter. Joint Task Force on Practice Parameters, the American Academy of Allergy, Asthma and Immunology, and the Joint Council of Allergy, Asthma and Immunology. Ann Allergy Asthma Immunol. 1999;83:665–700.

338. Mustafa SS. Anaphylaxis. In: Kaliner MA, editor. Medscape. http://emedicine.medscape.com/article/135065-overview#showall. Accessed 30 June 2016.

339. Annè S, Reisman RE. Risk of administering cephalosporin antibiotics to patients with histories of penicillin allergy. Ann Allergy Asthma Immunol. 1995;74(2):167–70.

340. Daulat S, Solensky R, Earl HS, Casey W, Gruchalla RS. Safety of cephalosporin administration to patients with histories of penicillin allergy. J Allergy Clin Immunol. 2004;113(6):1220–2.

341. Mertes PM, Malinovsky JM, Jouffroy L, et al. Reducing the risk of anaphylaxis during anesthesia: 2011 updated guidelines for clinical practice. J Investig Allergol Clin Immunol. 2011;21(6):442–53.

342. ten Holder SM, Joy MS, Falk RJ. Cutaneous and systemic manifestations of drug-induced vasculitis. Ann Pharmacother. 2002;36:130–47.

343. deShazo RD, Nelson HS. An approach to the patient with a history of local anesthetic hypersensitivity: experience with 90 patients. J Allergy Clin Immunol. 1979;63:387–94.

344. Moscicki RA, Sockin SM, Corsello BF, Ostro MG, Bloch KJ. Anaphylaxis during induction of general anesthesia: subsequent evaluation and management. J Allergy Clin Immunol. 1990;86:325–32.

345. Patterson R. Drug allergy and protocols for management of drug allergies. 2nd ed. Providence, RI: OceanSide Publications; 1995.

346. Hamilton RG, Adkinson NF Jr. Natural rubber latex skin testing reagents: safety and diagnostic accuracy of nonammoniated latex, ammoniated latex, and latex rubber glove extracts. J Allergy Clin Immunol. 1996;98:872–83.
347. Sogn DD, Evans R 3rd, Shepherd GM, Casale TB, Condemi J, Greenberger PA, et al. Results of the National Institute of Allergy and Infectious Diseases Collaborative Clinical Trial to test the predictive value of skin testing with major and minor penicillin derivatives in hospitalized adults. Arch Intern Med. 1992;152:1025–32.
348. Gruchalla RS, Sullivan TJ. In vivo and in vitro diagnosis of drug allergy. Immunol Allergy Clin N Am. 1991;11:595–610.
349. Schwartz LB. Tryptase, a mediator of human mast cells. J Allergy Clin Immunol. 1990;86:594–8.
350. Anne S, Reisman RE. Risk of administering cephalosporin antibiotics to patients with histories of penicillin allergy. Ann Allergy Asthma Immunol. 1995;74:167–70.
351. Adams LE, Hess EV. Drug-related lupus. Incidence, mechanisms and clinical implications. Drug Saf. 1991;6:431–49.
352. Craven NM. Management of toxic epidermal necrolysis. Hosp Med. 2000;61:778–81.
353. Sheffer AL, Austen KF. Exercise-induced anaphylaxis. J Allergy Clin Immunol. 1984;73(5 Pt 2):699–703.
354. Huynh PN. Exercise-Induced Anaphylaxis. In: Jyonouchi H, editor. Medscape. http://emedicine.medscape.com/article/886641-overview#showall. Accessed 2 July 2016.
355. Sheffer AL, Austen KF. Exercise-induced anaphylaxis. J Allergy Clin Immunol. 1980;66(2):106–11.
356. Shadick NA, Liang MH, Partridge AJ, et al. The natural history of exercise-induced anaphylaxis: survey results from a 10-year follow-up study. J Allergy Clin Immunol. 1999;104(1):123–7.
357. Aihara Y, Takahashi Y, Kotoyori T, et al. Frequency of food-dependent, exercise-induced anaphylaxis in Japanese junior-high-school students. J Allergy Clin Immunol. 2001;108(6):1035–9. https://doi.org/10.1067/mai.2001.119914.
358. Fiocchi A, Mirri GP, Santini I, Bernardo L, Ottoboni F, Riva E. Exercise-induced anaphylaxis after food contaminant ingestion in double-blinded, placebo-controlled, food-exercise challenge. J Allergy Clin Immunol. 1997;100(3):424–5.
359. Sanchez-Borges M, Iraola V, Fernandez-Caldas E, et al. Dust mite ingestion-associated, exercise-induced anaphylaxis. J Allergy Clin Immunol. 2007;120(3):714–6.
360. Longley S, Panush RS. Familial exercise-induced anaphylaxis. Ann Allergy. 1987;58(4):257–9.

361. Grant JA, Farnam J, Lord RA, Thueson DO, Lett-Brown MA, Wallfisch H. Familial exercise-induced anaphylaxis. Ann Allergy. 1985;54(1):35–8.

362. Maulitz RM, Pratt DS, Schocket AL. Exercise-induced anaphylactic reaction to shellfish. J Allergy Clin Immunol. 1979;63:433–4. https://doi.org/10.1016/0091-6749(79)90218-5.

363. Kidd JM III, Cohen SH, Sosman AJ, et al. Food-dependent exercise-induced anaphylaxis. J Allergy Clin Immunol. 1983;71:407–11. https://doi.org/10.1016/0091-6749(83)90070-2.

364. Barg W, Medrala W, Wolanczyk-Medrala A. Exercise-induced anaphylaxis: an update on diagnosis and treatment. Curr Allergy Asthma Rep. 2011;11(1):45–51.

365. Toit G. Food-dependent exercise-induced anaphylaxis in childhood. Pediatr Allergy Immunol. 2007;18:455–63. https://doi.org/10.1111/j.1399-3038.2007.00599.x.

366. Tanaka S. An epidemiological survey on food-dependent exercise-induced anaphylaxis in kindergartners, schoolchildren and junior high school students. Asia Pac J Public Health. 1994;7(1):26–30.

367. Ansley L, Bonini M, Delgado L, Del Giacco S, Du Toit G, Khaitov M, et al. Pathophysiological mechanisms of exercise-induced anaphylaxis: an EAACI position statement. Allergy. 2015;70(10):1212–21.

368. Lewis J, Lieberman P, Treadwell G, Erffmeyer J. Exercise-induced urticaria, angioedema, and anaphylactoid episodes. J Allergy Clin Immunol. 1981;68(6):432–7.

369. Schwartz HJ. Elevated serum tryptase in exercise-induced anaphylaxis. J Allergy Clin Immunol. 1995;95(4):917–9.

370. Casale TB, Bowman S, Kaliner M. Induction of human cutaneous mast cell degranulation by opiates and endogenous opioid peptides: evidence for opiate and nonopiate receptor participation. J Allergy Clin Immunol. 1984;73(6):775–81.

371. Hanakawa Y, Tohyama M, Shirakata Y, Murakami S, Hashimoto K. Food-dependent exercise-induced anaphylaxis: a case related to the amount of food allergen ingested. Br J Dermatol. 1998;138(5):898–900.

372. Heyman M. Gut barrier dysfunction in food allergy. Eur J Gastroenterol Hepatol. 2005;17(12):1279–85.

373. Fukutomi O, Kondo N, Agata H, et al. Abnormal responses of the autonomic nervous system in food-dependent exercise-induced anaphylaxis. Ann Allergy. 1992;68(5):438–45.

374. Palosuo K, Varjonen E, Nurkkala J, Kalkkinen N, Harvima R, Reunala T. Transglutaminase-mediated cross-linking of a peptic fraction of omega-5 gliadin enhances IgE reactivity in

wheat-dependent, exercise-induced anaphylaxis. J Allergy Clin Immunol. 2003;111(6):1386–92.

375. Shreffler WG, Lencer DA, Bardina L, Sampson HA. IgE and IgG4 epitope mapping by microarray immunoassay reveals the diversity of immune response to the peanut allergen, Ara h 2. J Allergy Clin Immunol. 2005;116(4):893–9.

376. Cooper DM, Radom-Aizik S, Schwindt C, Zaldivar F Jr. Dangerous exercise: lessons learned from dysregulated inflammatory responses to physical activity. J Appl Physiol. 2007;103(2):700–9.

377. Barg W, Wolanczyk-Medrala A, Obojski A, et al. Food-dependent exercise-induced anaphylaxis: possible impact of increased basophil histamine releasability in hyperosmolar conditions. J Investig Allergol Clin Immunol. 2008;18(4):312–5.

378. Wanderer AA. Cold urticaria syndromes: historical background, diagnostic classification, clinical and laboratory characteristics, pathogenesis, and management. J Allergy Clin Immunol. 1990;85(6):965–81.

379. Valent P. Diagnostic evaluation and classification of mastocytosis. Immunol Allergy Clin N Am. 2006;26(3):515–34.

380. Cicardi M, Agostoni A. Hereditary angioedema. N Engl J Med. 1996;334(25):1666–7.

381. Agostoni A, Aygoren-Pursun E, Binkley KE, et al. Hereditary and acquired angioedema: problems and progress: proceedings of the third C1 esterase inhibitor deficiency workshop and beyond. J Allergy Clin Immunol. 2004;114(3 Suppl):S51–131.

382. Feldweg AM. Exercise-induced anaphylaxis: management and prognosis. In: Kelso JM, TePas E, editors. UpToDate. 2016. http://www.uptodate.com/contents/exercise-induced-anaphylaxis-management-and-prognosis. Accessed 3 July 2016.

383. Juji F, Suko M. Effectiveness of disodium cromoglycate in food-dependent, exercise-induced anaphylaxis: a case report. Ann Allergy. 1994;72:452.

384. Sugimura T, Tananari Y, Ozaki Y, et al. Effect of oral sodium cromoglycate in 2 children with food-dependent exercise-induced anaphylaxis (FDEIA). Clin Pediatr (Phila). 2009;48:945.

385. Aihara Y, Kotoyori T, Takahashi Y, et al. The necessity for dual food intake to provoke food-dependent exercise-induced anaphylaxis (FEIAn): a case report of FEIAn with simultaneous intake of wheat and umeboshi. J Allergy Clin Immunol. 2001;107:1100.

386. Ueno M, Adachi A, Shimoura S, et al. A case of wheat-dependent exercise-induced anaphylaxis controlled by sodium chromoglycate, but not controlled by misoprostol. J Environ Dermatol Cutan Allergol. 2008;2:118.

387. Takahashi A, Nakajima K, Ikeda M, et al. Pre-treatment with misoprostol prevents food-dependent exercise-induced anaphylaxis (FDEIA). Int J Dermatol. 2011;50:237.

388. Inoue Y, Adachi A, Ueno M, et al. The inhibition effect of a synthetic analogue of prostaglandin E1 to the provocation by aspirin in the patients of WDEIA. Arerugi. 2009;58:1418.

389. Bray SM, Fajt ML, Petrov AA. Successful treatment of exercise-induced anaphylaxis with omalizumab. Ann Allergy Asthma Immunol. 2012;109:281.

390. Nutter AF. Contact urticaria to rubber. Br J Dermatol. 1979;101:597–8.

391. Gelfand DW. Barium enemas, latex balloons, and anaphylactic reactions. AJR Am J Roentgenol. 1991;156:1–2.

392. Turjanmaa K. Incidence of immediate allergy to latex gloves in hospital personnel. Contact Dermatitis. 1987;17:270–5.

393. Sussman G, Drouin MA, Hargreave FE, Douglas A, Turjanmaa K. Natural Rubber Latex Allergy. http://www.allergyfoundation.ca/index.php?page=64. Accessed 4 July 2016.

394. Reddy S. Latex Allergy. Am Fam Physician. 1998;57(1):93–100. http://www.aafp.org/afp/1998/0101/p93.html. Accessed 4 July 2016.

395. Conde-Salazar L, del Rio E, Guimaraens D, Gonzalez Domingo A. Type IV allergy to rubber additives: a 10-year study of 686 cases. J Am Acad Dermatol. 1993;29(2 Pt 1):176–80.

396. Beezhold D, Beck WC. Surgical glove powders bind latex antigens. Arch Surg. 1992;127:1354–7.

397. Alenius H, Makinen-Kiljunen S, Turjanmaa K, Palosuo T, Reunala T. Allergen and protein content of latex gloves. Ann Allergy. 1994;73:315–20.

398. Swanson MC, Bubak ME, Hunt LW, Yunginger JW, Warner MA, Read CE. Quantification of occupational latex aeroallergens in a medical center. J Allergy Clin Immunol. 1994;94(3 Pt 1):445–51.

399. Behrman AJ. Latex allergy. In: Schraga ED, editor. Medscape. http://emedicine.medscape.com/article/756632-overview. Accessed 4 July 2016.

400. Ahmed SM, Aw TC, Adisesh A. Toxicological and immunological aspects of occupational latex allergy. Toxicol Rev. 2004;23(2):123–34.

401. Jackson EM, Arnette JA, Martin ML, Tahir WM, Frost-Arner L, Edlich RF. A global inventory of hospitals using powder-free gloves: a search for principled medical leadership. J Emerg Med. 2000;18(2):241–6.

402. Ahmed DD, Sobczak SC, Yunginger JW. Occupational allergies caused by latex. Immunol Allergy Clin N Am. 2003;23(2):205–19.

403. Occupational Safety and Health Administration. Latex allergy. US Department of Labor. http://www.osha.gov/SLTC/latexallergy/index.html. Accessed 28 June 2013.
404. Dorevitch S, Forst L. The occupational hazards of emergency physicians. Am J Emerg Med. 2000;18(3):300–11.
405. Fein JA, Selbst SM, Pawlowski NA. Latex allergy in pediatric emergency department personnel. Pediatr Emerg Care. 1996;12(1):6–9.
406. Galindo MJ, Quirce S, Garcia OL. Latex allergy in primary care providers. J Investig Allergol Clin Immunol. 2011;21(6):459–65.
407. Schottler J, Vogel LC, Sturm P. Spinal cord injuries in young children: a review of children injured at 5 years of age and younger. Dev Med Child Neurol. 2012;54(12):1138–43.
408. Goldberg H, Aharony S, Levy Y, Sivan B, Baniel J, Ben Meir D. Low prevalence of latex allergy in children with spinal dysraphism in non-latex-free environment. J Pediatr Urol. 2016;12(1):52.e1–5.
409. Bernardini R, Catania P, Caffarelli C, et al. Perioperative latex allergy. Int J Immunopathol Pharmacol. 2011;24(3 Suppl):S55–60.
410. Caffarelli C, Stringari G, Miraglia Del Giudice M, Crisafulli G, Cardinale F, Peroni DG. Prevention of allergic reactions in anesthetized patients. Int J Immunopathol Pharmacol. 2011;24(3 Suppl):S91–9.
411. Dong SW, Mertes PM, Petitpain N, Hasdenteufel F, Malinovsky JM. Hypersensitivity reactions during anesthesia. Results from the ninth French survey (2005-2007). Minerva Anestesiol. 2012;78(8):868–78.
412. Thong BY, Yeow-Chan. Anaphylaxis during surgical and interventional procedures. Ann Allergy Asthma Immunol. 2004;92(6):619–28. [Medline].
413. Marmo M, Sacerdoti C, Di Minno RM, Guarino I, Villani R, Di Lorio C. Anaphylactic shock during hyperbaric oxygen therapy. Undersea Hyperb Med. 2012;39(1):613–6.
414. Taylor JS, Erkek E. Latex allergy: diagnosis and management. Dermatol Ther. 2004;17(4):289–301.
415. Hamilton RG, Peterson EL, Ownby DR. Clinical and laboratory-based methods in the diagnosis of natural rubber latex allergy. J Allergy Clin Immunol. 2002;110(2 Suppl):S47–56.
416. Accetta Pedersen DJ, Klancnik M, Elms N, et al. Analysis of available diagnostic tests for latex sensitization in an at-risk population. Ann Allergy Asthma Immunol. 2012;108(2):94–7.
417. Saulnier N, Nucera E, Altomonte G, Rizzi A, Pecora V, Aruanno A. Gene expression profiling of patients with latex and/or vegetable food allergy. Eur Rev Med Pharmacol Sci. 2012;16(9):1197–210.

418. United States Department of Health and Human Services, Public Health Service, Centers for Disease Control and Prevention, National Institute for Occupational Safety and Health. Preventing allergic reactions to natural rubber latex in the workplace. Cincinnati: Government Printing Office. 1997; NIOSH Publication No. 97–135.

419. Kwittken PL, Becker J, Oyefara B, Danziger R, Pawlowski N, Sweinberg S. Latex hypersensitivity reactions despite prophylaxis. Allergy Proc. 1992;13:123–7.

420. Food and Drug Administration. Natural rubber containing medical devices: user labeling. [Docket No. 96N-0119]. 21 CFR Part 801. Fed Regist. 1997;62:51021–30.

421. EpiPen. Who's at increased risk? https://www.epipen.com/what-is-anaphylaxis/what-causes-anaphylaxis/latex-allergy. Accessed 4 July 2016.

422. Crump VA. Idiopathic anaphylaxis: an update. http://www.allergyclinic.co.nz/idiopathic_anaphylaxis.aspx. Accessed 8 July 2016.

423. Bacal E, Patterson R, et al. Evaluation of severe anaphylactic reactions. Clin Allergy. 1978;8:295–309.

424. Grammer LC. Idiopathic anaphylaxis. In: Kelso JM, Feldweg AM, editors. Up to Date. http://021081h21.y.http.www.uptodate.com.proxy.kirikkale-elibrary.com/contents/idiopathic-anaphylaxis?source=search_result&search=Idiopathic+anaphyl axis&selectedTitle=1~23. Accessed 8 July 2016.

425. Lenchner K, Grammer LC. A current review of idiopathic anaphylaxis. Curr Opin Allergy Clin Immunol. 2003;3(4):305–11. http://www.medscape.com/viewarticle/460702_4. Accessed 8 July 2016.

426. Sampson HA, Mendelson L, Rosen JP. Fatal and near-fatal anaphylaxis to food in children and adolescents. N Engl J Med. 1992;327:380–4.

427. Kemp SF, Lockey RF, Wolf BL, Lieberman P. Anaphylaxis, a review of 266 cases. Arch Intern Med. 1995;155:1749–54.

428. Ditto AM, Harris KE, Krasnick J, Miller MA, Patterson R. Idiopathic anaphylaxis: a series of 335 cases. Ann Allergy Asthma Immunol. 1996;77:285–91.

429. Ditto AM, Krasnick J, Greenberger PA, Kelly KJ, McGrath K, Patterson R. Pediatric idiopathic anaphylaxis: experience with 22 patients. J Allergy Clin Immunol. 1997;100:320–6.

430. Greenberger PA. Idiopathic anaphylaxis. Immunol Allergy Clin N Am. 2007;27:273–93.

431. Tejedor Alonso MA, Sastre DJ, Sanchez-Hernandez JJ, et al. Idiopathic anaphylaxis: a descriptive study of 81 patients in Spain. Ann Allergy Asthma Immunol. 2002;88:313–8.

432. Webb LM, Lieberman P. Anaphylaxis: a review of 601 cases. Ann Allergy Asthma Immunol. 2006;97:39–43.

433. Patterson R, Hogan MB, Yarnold PR, Harris KE. Idiopathic anaphylaxis. An attempt to estimate the incidence in the United States. Arch Intern Med. 1995;155:869–71.
434. Shanmugam G, Schwartz LB, Khan DA. Prolonged elevation of tryptase in idiopathic anaphylaxis. J Allergy Clin Immunol. 2006;117:950–1.
435. Müller UR. Elevated baseline serum tryptase, mastocytosis and anaphylaxis. Clin Exp Allergy. 2009;39:620–2.
436. Brockow K, Jofer C, Behrendt H, Ring J. Anaphylaxis in patients with mastocytosis: a study on history, clinical features and risk factors in 120 patients. Allergy. 2008;63:226–32.
437. Akin C, Scott LM, Kocabas CN, et al. Demonstration of an aberrant mast-cell population with clonal markers in a subset of patients with "idiopathic" anaphylaxis. Blood. 2007;110:2331–3.
438. Grammer LC, Shaughnessy MA, Harris KE, Goolsby CL. Lymphocyte subsets and activation markers in patients with acute episodes of idiopathic anaphylaxis. Ann Allergy Asthma Immunol. 2000;85:368–71.
439. Howell DL, Jacobs C, Metz G, et al. Molecular profiling distinguishes patients with active idiopathic anaphylaxis from normal volunteers and reveals novel aspects of disease biology. J Allergy Clin Immunol. 2009;123:S150. Abstract.
440. Tanus T, et al. Serum Tryptase in idiopathic anaphylaxis a case report and review of the literature. Ann Emergency Med. 1994;24:104–7.
441. Ortolani C, Ispano M, Pastorello EA, Ansaloni R, Magri GC. Comparison of results of skin prick tests (with fresh foods and commercial food extracts) and RAST in 100 patients with oral allergy syndrome. J Allergy Clin Immunol. 1989;83:683–90.
442. Greenberger PA, Lieberman P. Idiopathic anaphylaxis. J Allergy Clin Immunol Pract. 2014;2(3):243–50; quiz 251. https://doi.org/10.1016/j.jaip.2014.02.012; Epub 2014 Apr 6.
443. Stallings AP, Platts-Mills TAE, Oliveira WM, Workman L, James HR, et al. Galactose-a-1,3-galactose and delayed anaphylaxis, angioedema, and urticarial in children. Pediatrics. 2013;1341:e1545–52.
444. Commins SP, Platts-Mills TA. Anaphylaxis syndromes related to a new mammalian cross-reactive carbohydrate determinant. J Allergy Clin Immunol. 2009;124:652–7.
445. Valent P, Akin C, Arock M, Brockow K, Butterfield JH, Carter MC, et al. Definitions, criteria and global classifications of mast cell disorders with special reference to mast cell activation syndromes: a consensus proposal. Int Arch Allergy Immunol. 2012;157:215–25.

446. Wiggins CA, Dykewicz MS, Patterson R. Idiopathic anaphylaxis: classification, evaluation, and treatment of 123 patients. J Allergy Clin Immunol. 1988;82:849–55.

447. Sampson HA, Mendelson L, Rosen JP. Fatal and near-fatal anaphylactic reactions to food in children and adolescents. N Engl J Med. 1992;327:380–4.

448. Bock SA, Muñoz-Furlong A, Sampson HA. Further fatalities caused by anaphylactic reactions to food, 2001-2006. J Allergy Clin Immunol. 2007;119:1016–8.

449. Pumphrey RS, Gowland MH. Further fatal allergic reactions to food in the United Kingdom, 1999-2006. J Allergy Clin Immunol. 2007;119:1018–9.

450. Greenberger PA, Rotskoff BD, Lifschultz B. Fatal anaphylaxis: postmortem findings and associated comorbid diseases. Ann Allergy Asthma Immunol. 2007;98:252–7.

451. Boxer MB, Greenberger PA, Patterson R. The impact of prednisone in life-threatening idiopathic anaphylaxis: reduction in acute episodes and medical costs. Ann Allergy. 1989;62:201–4.

452. Khan DA, Yocum MW. Clinical course of idiopathic anaphylaxis. Ann Allergy. 1994;73:370–4.

453. Patterson R, Fitzsimons EJ, Choy AC, Harris KE. Malignant and corticosteroid-dependent idiopathic anaphylaxis: successful responses to ketotifen. Ann Allergy Asthma Immunol. 1997;79:138–44.

454. Warrier P, Casale TB. Omalizumab in idiopathic anaphylaxis. Ann Allergy Asthma Immunol. 2009;102:257–8.

455. Demirtürk M, Gelincik A, Colakoğlu B, et al. Promising option in the prevention of idiopathic anaphylaxis: omalizumab. J Dermatol. 2012;39:552–4.

456. Borzutzky A, Morales PS, Mezzano V, et al. Induction of remission of idiopathic anaphylaxis with rituximab. J Allergy Clin Immunol. 2014;134:981–3.

Chapter 3
Pathophysiology of Anaphylaxis

3.1 Background

Exposure to an allergen to which the patient has been previously sensitised is necessary for anaphylaxis. Sensitisation involves the formation of IgE to epitopes on the allergen at initial exposure. B cells are responsible for the secretion of IgE, which is then bound by receptors for IgE (known as FcεRI receptors) with high affinity. These receptors are found on the outer membrane of mast cells and basophils [1–5]. When an allergen is represented, IgE binds and this causes FcεRI receptors to come close to each other and cross-link. Following cross-linkage, a number of tyrosine kinases (e.g. Lyn, syk, fyn) become active intracellularly, allowing both up- and down-regulation of the signalling cascade [3, 4]. The degranulation function of mast cells is dependent upon the influx of calcium to the cell, a process which can be facilitated or inhibited through intracellular signalling mechanisms [3, 6, 7]. Both mast cells and basophils form chemical signalling molecules in advance which can then be released upon demand. These stored molecules include histamine, heparin, tryptase, chymase, and tumour necrosis factor alpha (TNFα). The cells can also secrete inflammatory mediator substances such as platelet-activating factor, nitric oxide, TNFα, the products of the arachidonic acid cycle involving

© Springer Nature Switzerland AG 2020   163
C. Cingi, N. B. Muluk, *Quick Guide to Anaphylaxis*,
https://doi.org/10.1007/978-3-030-33639-4_3

cyclo-oxygenase (PGD2), and those involving lipoxygenase (in particular the leukotrienes LTC4, LTD4, and LTE4), but these are freshly synthesised rather than stored. Interleukins 4, 5, 13 plus GM-CSF may continue to be manufactured by the cell for some hours following exposure [6, 8].

3.2   Triggers for Anaphylactic Reactions

A number of countries share the feature that anaphylaxis is most commonly triggered by food, in particular groundnuts, tree nuts, shellfish, fish, milk, egg, and sesame [9–11]. It is, nonetheless, of note that there are differences between different geographical regions, and for some countries the triggers differ. Common triggers in this second group include chestnuts, rice, buckwheat, or chickpeas [12]. All foods have the potential to cause ana-phylaxis, and certain foods, which previously were considered non-allergenic, have now turned out to be triggers, for example, quinoa [13], dragon fruit [14], and certain uncooked red meat products where carbohydrates play a role [15]. Triggering food-stuffs may be latent, such as where different foods have been substituted, where there is cross-reactivity, and where foods have touched each other [11]. Ingredients added to foodstuffs, for example, some spices, gums of vegetable origin and colours, such as cochineal, can also act as triggers. If food is contami-nated with dust mites [16], or parasites (e.g. the nematode worm *Anisarkis simplex*, which infects fish caught at sea), these events may also explain the anaphylaxis [17, 18].

   Anaphylaxis caused by drugs is possible across the entire age range although its peak occurrence is in middle age and older life. The anti-microbials, in particular beta-lactam containing compounds, the NSAIDs (aspirin, ibuprofen, others) and chemo-therapy drugs are frequently found to be the cause of anaphylaxis [9, 10, 19–25]. Drugs which have recently been discovered to be triggers for anaphylaxis have included loperamide [22], some contaminating substances found in drugs, such as over-sulphated chondroitin sulphate in heparin [23] and drugs which do not immediately spring to mind as potential causes, for example, vitamin or dietary supplements such as folic acid [24] and herbal medicines [25]. There is a developing awareness that drugs used perioperatively, as radiological contrast (iodine), and as dyes for medical use can act as triggers, including outside a hospital setting. Biologics known to cause anaphylaxis include the monoclonal antibodies cetuximab, infliximab, and omalizumab [26–28] and allergens deliberately employed in desensitising immunotherapeutic regimes [29, 30]. Vaccines used in the prevention of infectious disease only rarely cause anaphylaxis. Where this has occurred, the vaccine itself is not usually implicated [31–34], instead excipients that contain protein, for example, gelatin or eggs are typically found to be responsible, as, from time to time are other excipients, such as dextran [18, 31, 34].

Venoms injected by insects through their stings, in particular insects of the order Hymenoptera (Vespid family—Yellow jackets, yellow- and white-faced hornets, and paper wasps or Formicid family—i.e. ants [35–37]) can provoke an anaphylactic reaction. In addition, but rather less frequently, saliva injected when insects bite (flies, mosquitoes, ticks, kissing bugs, and caterpillars) may set off an anaphylactic episode [18, 37–40].

The campaign to stop anaphylaxis due to natural rubber latex has up to now focused on the usage in healthcare environments and has achieved some success. In the wider community, though, there are still reports coming through from time to time indicating that anaphylaxis is occurring as a result of exposure to gloves made from latex, condoms, racket handles, balloons, and sandpits where the floor is formed from latex, babies' dummies, and feeding bottle nipples. Since a number of foodstuffs can cross-react with a latex allergy (bananas, kiwis, papayas, avocados, potatoes, and tomatoes are of this kind), these, too, may provoke an anaphylactic reaction in a latex-sensitised patient [41]. Allergenic substances encountered at work [10], seminal fluid [42] and, on infrequent occasions, inhaled allergens, for example, animal dander [43] or pollen originating from grass, all may provoke anaphylaxis. It is probable that a degree of absorption into the circulation is occurring in these cases [18].

3.3   Pathophysiology

In the majority of cases, anaphylaxis is thought to occur as a result of mast cells and basophils becoming activated via immunoglobulin E cross-linkage and subsequent FcεRI aggregation. FcεRI is a receptor molecule which avidly binds IgE. Mast cells, with or without basophils, degranulate swiftly when activated, thereby releasing histamine, tryptase, carboxy-peptidase A, and proteoglycans. Phospholipase A2 (PLA2), which occurs later in the cascade, is forward-activated, as are the cyclo-oxygenases and lipoxygenases. These last two metabolise arachidonic acid to produce prostaglandins, leucotrienes, and platelet-activating factor (PAF). Tumour necrosis factor alpha (TNF α) is a cytokine in the inflammatory cascade that is synthesised in advance and released early on as well as acting in concert at a later stage with other cytokines and chemokines. A large number of these signalling molecules are implicated in the pathophysiology of anaphylaxis. The actions of histamine include causing blood vessels to dilate and to become more permeable, raising the heart rate, increasing contractility of the heart, and provoking secretion from glands. Prostaglandin D2 causes the bronchi to constrict, increases the tone in pulmonary and coronary blood vessels, and causes dilation of the blood vessels in the periphery. The effect of leucotrienes is to constrict the bronchi, enhance permeability of vessels, and cause airways to alter their cellular structure. PAF release causes marked bronchial constriction and in addition enhances the porosity of endothelium. TNF alpha causes neutrophils to become activated, orchestrates a response from other cells, and promotes the synthesis of chemokines [44]. Therefore, multiple different effects on physiology operating at the same time and in a synergistic fashion produce the pathological anaphylactic response. Anaphylaxis itself clinically is seen as a generalised urticaria action with angioedema, spasm of the bronchitis, and other symptoms related to breathing, low blood pressure, transient loss of consciousness, and other circulating symptoms. The gut is also affected, leading to nausea sensations, abdominal, and other gastrointestinal symptoms. Anaphylaxis may also happen in two distinct phases with a prolonged duration [3].

There are instances documented of anaphylaxis having taken place through a mechanism independent of IgE, amongst which the possibility of anaphylatoxins, which are part of the complement pathway, being activated, the release of neuropeptides, the production of immuno complexes, cytotoxicity, the activation of T cells, or possibly several effects working together, have been proposed as an explanation for non-IgE-mediated anaphylaxis [3, 45]. A second anaphylactic pathway has newly been delineated using mice as a model organism. The first pathway depends upon immunoglobulin E, aggregation of FCεRI receptors, and mast cells degranulating, with histamine and PAF being released. The second pathway uses the IgG molecule and its receptor, FcγRIII, and in this case it is PAF rather than histamine which plays the key role [46–50]. An advantage of murine models of mast cell function is that gene knockout variance can be used to assess how particular genes are involved in the signal cascade in general. In humans, the majority of anaphylactic reactions occur through IgE, but evidence does exist pointing to the involvement of IgG or systems other than the immune system. These reactions are referred to as anaphylactoid [50]. How IgG functions to produce anaphylaxis in Man is not explored in the literature or, indeed, adequately understood [3, 51].

Accepted practice has been to restrict the meaning of the term anaphylaxis to where IgE is the principal mediator. Anaphylactoid is then applied to reactions not mediated through IgE. In clinical practice, these reactions appear the same. The World Allergy Organization recommends that the terms "anaphylactic" and "anaphylactoid" be replaced with "immunologic" and "non-immunologic" anaphylaxis. Immunologic anaphylaxis therefore corresponds to anaphylaxis occurring through the medium of IgE or through IgG and the formation of immune complexes and the complement cascade, whilst non-immunologic anaphylaxis involves acute degranulation of mast cells and basophils but no immunoglobulin involvement [52].

Physiologically speaking, the anaphylaxis cascade triggers smooth muscles to contract within the respiratory tree and the gut, blood vessels to dilate, endothelial permeability to increase, and sensory nerve endings to be stimulated. It is the presence of additional mucus and the heightened tone of bronchial smooth muscle, together with oedema within the airways which explains the symptomatic phenomenology of anaphylaxis [53].

Symptoms affecting the circulatory system are result of lower tone in the vasculature and loss of fluid from the capillaries. Low blood pressure, rhythmic abnormalities of the heart, loss of consciousness, and shock may occur as a result of loss of circulating volume, vasodilation, and problems with the functioning of the cardiac muscle. Within a 10-min space, 35% of the volume contained within the circulation may move outside the blood vessels [53].

These physiological alterations cause all or a portion of the symptoms typically seen in anaphylactic reactions. Reddening of the skin, hives and angioedema, itching, spasm of the bronchitis, swelling within the larynx, griping pains with the urge to vomit and actual vomiting, loose and watery stools, and *angor animi*. Other effects include a watery nasal discharge, hoarseness, metallic taste in the mouth, uterine cramping, dizziness, and headaches [53].

There are a number of other signalling molecules which set into action other inflammatory pathways. Such mediators include the neutral proteases, tryptase and chymase, proteoglycans (including heparin and chondroitin sulphate), the cytokines, and chemokines. Different pathways are activated by these signal molecules such as the kallikrein-kinin system, complement cascade and pathways leading to coagulation. The way in which, and the degree to which, anaphylaxis develops is a function of how responsive cellular mediators are to these molecules [53].

During the first stage of anaphylaxis, interleukins 4 and 13 are significant in orchestrating the production of antibody and the recruitment of cells of the inflammatory system. Whilst the roles in humans have not been experimentally confirmed, in mice, anaphylaxis hinges upon a transcription factor, STAT-6 (signal transducer and activator of transcription 6) being activated by interleukins 4 and 13 via IL-4Rα [50]. Eosinophils play both pro-inflammatory and anti-inflammatory roles. They are pro-inflammatory when they degranulate with the release of cytotoxic messenger molecules. They are anti-inflammatory when they break down molecules which affect the tone within blood vessels [53].

There are some further signalling molecules of importance. These include prostaglandin D2 and leukotriene B4, which are metabolised from lipid precursors, PAF and cysteinyl leukotrienes, for example, LTC4, LTD4, and LTE4. These all have pro-inflammatory actions in the context of anaphylaxis [53].

Within tightly controlled experiments, administering histamine is enough on its own to give rise to the majority of anaphylactic symptoms. Histamine operates through two receptors, H1 and H2 [53].

Both histamine receptor subtypes 1 and 2 control the dilation of blood vessels, the lowering of blood pressure, and the reddening of the skin. The constriction of coronary artery vessels, the increased pulse rate, the enhanced degree to which vessels are permeable, itching, spasm of the bronchi, and watery nasal discharge all occur as a result of H1 receptors alone. H2 receptors, on the other hand, increase the degree to which the atria and ventricles contract, alter the rate at which the atria contract, and cause coronary blood vessels to dilate. In experiments involving dogs, H3 receptors seemingly play a role on how the circulatory system responds to norepinephrine. How big a role H3 receptors play in humans is currently not known [53].

3.3.1 Immunologic Reactions Mediated Through IgE

The classical examples of anaphylactic reaction occurring through the medium of IgE are those occurring in drug, food, and insect venom allergies. In all parts of the industrialised world, food allergies are observed [54]. Within the USA, it is estimated that four million individuals have an allergy to food which can be verified. Research originating from Australia revealed that at least 10% of children aged 1 year had an allergy to some type of food occurring through the medium of IgE and shown to exist through a formal food challenge [55]. In Montréal, a prevalence of 1.5% for groundnut allergy was found in children attending early elementary school. Amongst cases of anaphylaxis which occur outside a hospital, food allergy is considered the most frequent cause [53].

There are particular foods which are associated with the greater likelihood of stimulating an IgE response. This group of foods is the same across all ages and encompasses tree nuts, groundnuts, fish, and shellfish. In children, additionally cows' milk, eggs, wheat, and soya are pro-allergenic [53].

A case series of lethal anaphylaxis secondary to food allergy concluded that the most probable allergen was peanut in 62% of the deaths. A person with a peanut sensitivity may show a response even to as low an amount as 100 µg of groundnut protein, as has been revealed in formal food challenges where a placebo was also administered [56]. The Rochester Epidemiology Project confirmed what had earlier been stated by researchers, viz. that food allergies accounted for more cases of anaphylaxis than any other cause, perhaps up to one third of such reactions [57].

Traditionally, past history of allergy to eggs involving production of specific IgE was considered a reason not to give the annual influenza vaccination. Until fairly recently, patients known to be allergic to eggs were vaccinated for influenza, but usually by following a procedure in which the dose was gradually escalated, or after cutaneous testing of the vaccine itself. Proof that patients who are allergic to eggs can be given vaccination for influenza without increasing the risk of a generalised allergic reaction as compared to the background risk is lacking; hence, the latest edition of the vaccination guidelines proposed that anyone with an allergy to eggs should receive the vaccine for influenza as a single dose. In addition, cutaneous testing is not beneficial due to a lack of evidence that this procedure allows the stratification of risk amongst individuals receiving the vaccination [58, 59].

From time to time, food poisoning as a result of eating scombroid fish may closely resemble anaphylaxis secondary to food allergy. This is because bacteria which are found in decaying fish are a source of enzymes that can decarboxylase histamine, thereby producing amines with biological action such as histamine and cis-urocanic acid, both of which can trigger mast cells to degranulate [53].

The majority of drug allergies in the USA (i.e. those mediated through IgE) are due to penicillin or the other beta-lactams. Intravenous administration of penicillin or antibiotic of cephalosporin kind produces an anaphylactic reaction in around one case in 5000 [53].

Within the body, penicillin is mostly metabolised to benzyl-penicilloyl, but also a number of other molecules. These are the source of allergies. Penicillin and the metabolites thereof are so small that they can only be reacted to by the immune system when they have been bound to carrier proteins. They are therefore termed haptens. There is a possibility of cross-reactivity between penicillins and other beta-lactams. First-generation, older type cephalosporins, such as cephalothin, cefadroxil, and cephalozin generally provoke hypersensitivities with greater frequency than newer cephalosporins, such as cefprozil, cefuroxime, ceftazidime, or ceftriaxone. The explanation for this relates to the greater similarity of the side-chain in first-generation agents to the antigenic determinants of penicillin. The side-chain was removed from second- and third- generation agents [53].

Multiple different drugs have been linked to allergic type anaphylaxis although with less frequency than the beta-lactams. For surgical patients, anaphylactic reactions will most likely occur secondary to the use of muscle relaxants. However, hypnotics, antibiotics, opioids, colloids, and other agents also share the capability of inducing anaphylaxis. Formerly, during the 1980s, when concerns about HIV and hepatitis B and C were at their peak, latex was widely used for barrier protection in clinical settings and this resulted in a peak in latex allergy occurrences. Since that date, non-latex materials have increased in use and therefore allergy rates are falling. A characteristic of anaphylaxis caused by latex perioperatively is that such reactions are more common whilst anaesthesia is being maintained, whereas anaphylaxis secondary to other substances is most likely to happen whilst anaesthesia is being induced. Inhalational anaesthetics are known to be hepatotoxic through an immune mechanism, but have not been reported as the cause of anaphylaxis [60].

Stings by Hymenoptera insects commonly provoke both allergic reactions in general and anaphylaxis in particular. Within the general American population, the prevalence of generalised reaction following a sting is between 0.5 and 3% [61]. Venom from such insects causes a mortality of under 100 annually in the USA. It is much more frequent to observe localised reactions with hives but no other signs of anaphylaxis than frank anaphylaxis when a patient has been stung. Suffers from systemic urticaria run an increased risk of developing anaphylaxis stung in the future, but how severe a local reaction is has no bearing on the anaphylactic risk profile [53].

3.3.2 Immune-Mediated Reactions to Aspirin, NSAIDs, and ACE Inhibitors

Traditionally, hypersensitive reactions to aspirin or the NSAIDs have been treated differently from true drug allergies, dependent as there are on IgE, because of a supposedly different pathophysiological mechanism, involving arachidonic acid. However, skin reactions occurring on their own to aspirin or the NSAIDs, and spasm of the bronchi in patients with asthma who are aspirin-sensitive, frequently associated with the development of polyps in the nose, do depend upon IgE. NSAIDs and aspirin block cyclo-oxygenase, thus inhibiting the prostanoid pathway, and leukotrienes are over-produced as a result through the 5-lipoxygenase pathway. Cross-reactions are frequent between aspirin and the majority of NSAIDs [53].

When anaphylaxis occurs with these medications, however, a different pathophysiological mechanism is responsible, one that seemingly fits better with the idea that IgE is a central actor.

In cases of genuine anaphylaxis, there does not seem to be any cross-reactivity between these drugs, which share the feature of cyclo-oxygenase inhibition. In addition, for anaphylaxis to occur, it appears that two exposures are required, hinting at a preceding sensitisation stage. One last piece of evidence is that it is unusual for cases of true anaphylaxis to occur in patients who already have asthma, nasal polyps, or hives [53].

3.3.3 Immune Reactions Occurring Through Mechanisms Other than IgE

The use of blood-derived products such as intravenous immuno-globulins, or animal-derived antisera, is associated with anaphylaxis, to an extent attributable to the action of the complement cascade. The complement cascade produces several molecules which can make mast cells and basophils degranulate [53].

An unusual form of anaphylaxis, that has two variants, is exercise-induced anaphylaxis. In the first variant, the consumption of food (e.g. wheat or celery) or medication (e.g. NSAIDs) within a short period before exercising is sufficient in itself to provoke an episode of anaphylaxis. Neither exercise alone nor the particular foods ingested are sufficient to provoke the symptoms [53]. In the second variant, anaphylaxis occurs from time to time during exercise, without food playing a role. Anaphylaxis is not an invariable consequence of the patient performing physically demanding activities. It is worthy of note that systemic mastocytosis, a disorder in which there are abnormally elevated levels of mast cells in several organs, can present as anaphylaxis. The risk of food and insect venom allergic reactions is raised in this group. It is widely suggested that alcohol, vancomycin, opioids, radiological contrast media, and other bioactive substances that can cause the degranulation of mast cells be avoided in systemic mastocytosis [53].

3.3.4   Reactions Not Mediated by the Immune System

Some drugs, including the opioids, dextran, protamine, and vancomycin, it is believed, may possess the ability to stimulate the release of signalling molecules from mast cells without immune involvement. In addition, some evidence points to the activation of diverse inflammatory pathways by dextrans and protamine. These pathways encompass the complement and coagulation cascades and the vasoactive kallikrein-kinin system [53].

Contrast materials used in radiology that are given intravenously can provoke anaphylactoid reactions that resemble anaphylaxis clinically and are managed identically. There is no association with previous exposure. Around 1–3 in 100 patients who are given hyperosmolar contrast media intravenously have a hypersensitivity response. For the most part, such reactions are mild and limited to urticaria, and few such reactions have resulted in death. The risk of dying from the use of radiological contrast has been calculated as 0.9 in 100,000 procedures [53].

The administration of histamine blockers or steroids prophylactically, together with the usage of lower molecular weight contrast media has diminished the rate of anaphylactoid reaction to around 0.5%. In patients who have previously had such a reaction, the risk of it occurring a second time is between 17 and 60%, and therefore such prophylactic treatment should be contemplated. Some settings permit only the use of the lower molecular weight contrast agents. Administering contrast should only occur where facilities (staff, drugs, emergency equipment) are suitable for emergency resuscitation. Consent needs to be obtained prior to the procedure [53].

Patients with known atopy for asthma have an enhanced risk of reacting. Patients who use beta-blockers are harder to treat for allergic reactions. However, being allergic to shellfish or iodine neither prevents the use of contrast media nor does it necessarily entail prophylactic treatment. Lower molecular weight contrast media available may be better, as is the case with all patients who have an allergy. Iodine allergy is a confusing term since iodine must be present in the body in trace amounts for health. Thus, an allergy to iodine cannot truly occur. Patients with a past history of iodine allergy typically have experienced either hypersensitivity to contrast, allergy to shellfish, or localised irritation following the use of povidine (betadine) [53].

Since contrast media as used to explore the genitourinary or gastrointestinal tracts, i.e. in contact with mucosal surfaces but not absorbed systemically, does not seem to provoke anaphylaxis, a documented allergy need not prevent their use in these applications [53].

3.4 Mechanisms of Anaphylaxis

Research into how mast cells become activated has been reported from in vitro studies (human plus other mammals) and in vivo at the tissue and whole animal levels. Very recent studies draw attention to the regulatory role of mast cells in how anaphylaxis develops. To understand the pathophysiology of anaphylaxis, recognition of how intracellular mechanisms cause mediator release is a vital step. It is through these intracellular signalling pathways that mast cells are able to degranulate at such speed, and arachidonic acid pathways to adapt to the production of lipid-based mediator substances, and the chemokines and cytokines eventually to be produced. Activating mast cells and triggering the release of chemical signals hinges on IgE binding to FCεRI. Once IgE is bound, there is aggregation of the receptors, which sets off a cascade of signals. FCεRI molecules contain regions known as immunoreceptor tyrosine-based activation motifs (ITAMs), rich in tyrosine residues. These sequences become phosphorylated through the action of tyrosine kinases belonging to the Src family, members of which include Lyn and Syk. Syk becomes part of a signalling complex and phosphorylates itself to promote further activity, in addition to being phosphorylated by the Lyn enzyme. Adaptor molecules which span the membrane are linked and following phosphorylation by the tyrosine kinases, activate the T-cell linker molecule (LAT) and the non-cell linker molecule (NTAL). These then supply scaffolding for interactions (directly or indirectly) with other adaptor molecules such as Grb2, Gads, Shc, and SLP76, the guanine nucleotide exchange factors and Sos and Vav (adaptor molecules), plus phospholipase Cγ (PLCγ) and PI3 kinase, which are the key enzymes in the signalling cascade. Once these last two enzymes have been activated, calcium sequestered intracellularly is released, and this leads to protein kinase C becoming active, an event that prompts mast cells to degranulate. The Ras-raf-mitogen-activated protein (MAP) kinase pathway operates as a result of the action of Sos and Vav. PLA2 is thereby activated, arachidonic acid synthesised, and lipid-based mediators are generated and released. AP-1, NFAT (nuclear factor of activated T cells), and NF-κB are transcription factors whose activation leads to the synthesis of cytokines and chemokines. Fyn (tyrosine kinase) has an effect via a different signalling pathway by the phosphorylation of the adaptor protein Gab2, thereby activating PI3K, Bruton's tyrosine kinase (Btk), PLCγ, and sphingosine kinase and increasing production of sphingosine-1-phosphate (S1P) [3, 62, 63].

Studies published within the last 12 months have emphasised the centrality of the tyrosine kinases in initially activating FCεRI and the way downstream events may regulate the formation of the signal complex. There are multiple points at which the signalling cascade is both up- and down-regulated. It is known that three tyrosine kinases are essential to transducing signals (Lyn, Syk, and Fyn); however, other enzymes of the same type are now emerging as of vital importance, for example, Hek, the role of which in positively regulating the degranulation of mast cells through inhibiting Lyn and phosphorylating FCεRI was demonstrated in genetically mutated mice in 2007 [64]. Lyn plays a role through phosphorylating tyrosine at the beginning when the signalling cascade is activated and its actions ensure the involvement of other proteins involved in regulation at a lower level in the cascade [62]. How intensely FCεRI was stimulated was proven to have a determining effect on the regulation of the signal cascade at its lower levels via activation of Lyn. The presence of stimuli classified as of low intensity, such as IgE in its monomer form, IgE simultaneously with anti-IgE, or IgE present but with low levels of antigen had a positive regulatory effect on how mast cells degranulated and produced cytokines, by lowering the activity of Lyn and preventing interaction with FCεRI. On the other hand, the situation in which a stimulus could be considered of high-intensity, such as abundant IgE and potent levels of antigen, led to a negative regulatory effect on mast cells by increasing the activity of Lyn and its interaction with FCεRI, plus an increase in the actions of Syk [3, 65].

Activated Fyn is the second mechanism whereby mast cells may degranulate in response to the actions of tyrosine kinases. The presence of Fyn is needed for mast cells to degranulate and produce cytokines, just as it is known that Lyn plays a central role in the up- and down-regulation of initial and later events within the signalling pathway in mast cells [66]. Gab2 (an adaptor molecule) is phosphorylated by Fyn, an event that triggers the aggregation of the signalling complex by the involvement of PI3K, PLCγ, Btk, and Vav [62]. Studies have newly been published in which the regulation of PI3K is discussed, with its concomitant effect of inhibiting anaphylaxis. A 2008 study revealed that RGS13, which belongs to the regulator of G protein signalling family (RGS), prevents the signal action of PI3K through forming a bond with the p85 regulatory subunit, thereby halting interaction with Gab2 and Grb2, which are proteins involved in scaffolding. RGS13 double knockout mice have upgraded mast cell degranulation and greater anaphylactic responses [3, 67].

References

1. Sampson HA, et al. Second symposium on the definition and management of anaphylaxis: summary report—Second National Institute of Allergy and Infectious Disease/Food Allergy and Anaphylaxis Network symposium. J Allergy Clin Immunol. 2006;117:391–7.
2. Simons FE. Anaphylaxis, killer allergy: long-term management in the community. J Allergy Clin Immunol. 2006;117:367–77.

3. Peavy RD, Metcalfe DD. Understanding the mechanisms of anaphylaxis. Curr Opin Allergy Clin Immunol. 2008;8(4):310–5. https://doi.org/10.1097/ACI.0b013e3283036a90.

4. Metcalfe DD, Peavy RD, Gilfillan AM. Mechanisms of mast cell signaling in anaphylaxis. J Allergy Clin Immunol. 2009;124:639–46; quiz 647–648.

5. Kalesnikoff J, Galli SJ. New developments in mast cell biology. Nat Immunol. 2008;9:1215–23.

6. Boden SR, Burks AW. Anaphylaxis: a history with emphasis on food allergy. Immunol Rev. 2011;242(1):247–57.

7. Bansal G, et al. Suppression of immunoglobulin E-mediated allergic responses by regulator of G protein signaling 13. Nat Immunol. 2008;9:73–80.

8. Brown SG. The pathophysiology of shock in anaphylaxis. Immunol Allergy Clin N Am. 2007;27:165–75. v.

9. Simons FER. Anaphylaxis: recent advances in assessment and treatment. J Allergy Clin Immunol. 2009;124:625–36.

10. Lieberman PL. Anaphylaxis. In: Adkinson Jr NF, Bochner BS, Busse WW, Holgate ST, Lemanske Jr RF, Simons FER, editors. Middleton's allergy: principles and practice. 7th ed. St. Louis: Mosby; 2009. p. 1027–49.

11. Sampson HA, Burks AW. Adverse reactions to foods. In: Adkinson Jr NF, Bochner BS, Busse WW, Holgate ST, Lemanske Jr RF, Simons FER, editors. Middleton's allergy: principles and practice. 7th ed. St. Louis: Mosby; 2009. p. 1139–67.

12. Shek LPC, Lee BW. Food allergy in Asia. Curr Opin Allergy Clin Immunol. 2006;6:197–201.

13. Astier C, Moneret-Vautrin DA, Puillandre E, Bihain BE. First case report of anaphylaxis to quinoa, a novel food in France. Allergy. 2009;64:819–20.

14. Kleinheinz A, Lepp U, Hausen BM, Petersen A, Becker WM. Anaphylactic reaction to (mixed) fruit juice containing dragon fruit. J Allergy Clin Immunol. 2009;124:841–2.

15. Commins SP, Satinover SM, Hosen J, Mozena J, Borish L, Lewis BD, et al. Delayed anaphylaxis, angioedema, or urticaria after consumption of red meat in patients with IgE antibodies specific for galactose-alpha-1,3-galactose. J Allergy Clin Immunol. 2009;123:426–33.

16. Sanchez-Borges M, Iraola V, Fernandez-Caldas E, Capriles-Hulett A, Caballero-Fonseca F. Dust mite ingestion-associated, exercise-induced anaphylaxis. J Allergy Clin Immunol. 2007;120:714–6.

17. Petithory JC. New data on anisakiasis. Bull Acad Natl Med. 2007;191:53–65.

18. Simons FER. Anaphylaxis. J Allergy Clin Immunol. 2010;125(2):S161–81.

19. Celik W, Pichler WJ, Adkinson NF Jr. Drug allergy. In: Adkinson Jr NF, Bochner BS, Busse WW, Holgate ST, Lemanske Jr RF, Simons FER, editors. Middleton's allergy: principles and practice. 7th ed. St. Louis: Mosby; 2009. p. 1205–26.

20. Novembre E, Mori F, Pucci N, Bernardini R, Romano A. Cefaclor anaphylaxis in children. Allergy. 2009;64:1233–5.

21. Berges-Gimeno M, Martin-Lazaro J. Allergic reactions to non-steroidal anti-inflammatory drugs: is newer better? Curr Allergy Asthma Rep. 2007;7:35–40.

22. Perez-Calderon R, Gonzalo-Garijo MA. Anaphylaxis due to loperamide. Allergy. 2004;59:369–70.

23. Kishimoto TK, Viswanathan K, Ganguly T, Elankumaran S, Smith S, Pelzer K, et al. Contaminated heparin associated with adverse clinical events and activation of the contact system. N Engl J Med. 2008;358:2457–67.

24. Nishitani N, Adachi A, Fukumoto T, Ueno M, Fujiwara N, Ogura K, et al. Folic acid-induced anaphylaxis showing cross-reactivity with methotrexate: a case report and review of the literature. Int J Dermatol. 2009;48:522–4.

25. Ji KM, Li M, Chen JJ, Zhan ZK, Liu ZG. Anaphylactic shock and lethal anaphylaxis caused by Houttuynia Cordata injection, a herbal treatment in China. Allergy. 2009;64:816–7.

26. Chung CH, Mirakhur B, Chan E, Le QT, Berlin J, Morse M, et al. Cetuximab-induced anaphylaxis and IgE specific for galactose-alpha-1,3-galactose. N Engl J Med. 2008;358:1109–17.

27. Cheifetz A, Smedley M, Martin S, Reiter M, Leone G, Mayer L, et al. The incidence and management of infusion reactions to infliximab: a large center experience. Am J Gastroenterol. 2003;98:1315–24.

28. Limb SL, Starke PR, Lee CE, Chowdhury BA. Delayed onset and protracted progression of anaphylaxis after omalizumab administration in patients with asthma. J Allergy Clin Immunol. 2007;120:1378–81.

29. Rezvani M, Bernstein DI. Anaphylactic reactions during immunotherapy. Immunol Allergy Clin N Am. 2007;27:295–307.

30. Rodriguez-Perez N, Ambriz-Moreno M, Canonica GW, Penagos M. Frequency of acute systemic reactions in patients with allergic rhinitis and asthma treated with sublingual immunotherapy. Ann Allergy Asthma Immunol. 2008;101:304–10.

31. Kelso JM, Li JT, Nicklas RA, Bernstein DI, Blessing-Moore J, Cox L, et al. Adverse reactions to vaccines. Ann Allergy Asthma Immunol. 2009;103(suppl):S1–S14.

32. Slade BA, Leidel L, Vellozzi C, Woo EJ, Hua W, Sutherland A, et al. Postlicensure safety surveillance for quadrivalent human papillomavirus recombinant vaccine. JAMA. 2009;302:750–7.

33. Erlewyn-Lajeunesse M, Brathwaite N, Lucas JSA, Warner JO. Recommendations for the administration of influenza vaccine in children allergic to egg. BMJ. 2009;339:b3680.
34. Zanoni G, Puccetti A, Dolcino M, Simone R, Peretti A, Ferro A, et al. Dextran-specific IgG response in hypersensitivity reactions to measles-mumps-rubella vaccine. J Allergy Clin Immunol. 2008;122:1233–5.
35. Golden DBK. Insect allergy. In: Adkinson Jr NF, Bochner BS, Busse WW, Holgate ST, Lemanske Jr RF, Simons FER, editors. Middleton's allergy: principles and practice. 7th ed. St. Louis: Mosby; 2009. p. 1005–17.
36. Bilo MB, Bonifazi F. The natural history and epidemiology of insect venom allergy: clinical implications. Clin Exp Allergy. 2009;39:1467–76.
37. Freeman TM. Clinical practice. Hypersensitivity to hymenoptera stings. N Engl J Med. 2004;351:1978–84.
38. Tankersley MS. The stinging impact of the imported fire ant. Curr Opin Allergy Clin Immunol. 2008;8:354–9.
39. Shek LPC, Ngiam NSP, Lee BW. Ant allergy in Asia and Australia. Curr Opin Allergy Clin Immunol. 2004;4:325–8.
40. Peng Z, Beckett AN, Engler RJ, Hoffman DR, Ott NL, Simons FER. Immune responses to mosquito saliva in 14 individuals with acute systemic allergic reactions to mosquito bites. J Allergy Clin Immunol. 2004;114:1189–94.
41. Yunginger JW. Natural rubber latex allergy. In: Adkinson Jr NF, Bochner BS, Busse WW, Holgate ST, Lemanske Jr RF, Simons FER, editors. Middleton's allergy: principles and practice. 7th ed. St. Louis: Mosby; 2009. p. 1019–26.
42. Basagana M, Bartolome B, Pastor C, Torres F, Alonso R, Vivanco F, et al. Allergy to human seminal fluid: cross-reactivity with dog dander. J Allergy Clin Immunol. 2008;121:233–9.
43. Gawlik R, Pitsch T. Allergy to horse. Ann Allergy Asthma Immunol. 2006;96:631.
44. Ogawa Y, Grant JA. Mediators of anaphylaxis. Immunol Allergy Clin N Am. 2007;27:249–60.
45. Simons FE, Frew AJ, Ansotegui IJ, et al. Risk assessment in anaphylaxis: current and future approaches. J Allergy Clin Immunol. 2007;120:S2–24.
46. Finkelman FD, Rothenberg ME, Brandt EB, et al. Molecular mechanisms of anaphylaxis: lessons from studies with murine models. J Allergy Clin Immunol. 2005;115:449–57.
47. Strait RT, Morris SC, Yang M, et al. Pathways of anaphylaxis in the mouse. J Allergy Clin Immunol. 2002;109:658–68.

48. Baeza ML, Zubeldia JM. Immunology of anaphylaxis: lessons from murine models. Curr Allergy Asthma Rep. 2007;7:49–55.
49. Nauta A, Knippels L, Garssen J, Redegeld F. Animal models of anaphylaxis. Curr Opin Allergy Clin Immunol. 2007;7:355–9.
50. Finkelman FD. Anaphylaxis: lessons from mouse models. J Allergy Clin Immunol. 2007;120(3):506–15; quiz 516–7.
51. Nieuwenhuizen N, Herbert DR, Lopata AL, Brombacher F. CD4+ T cell-specific deletion of IL-4 receptor alpha prevents ovalbumin-induced anaphylaxis by an IFN-gamma-dependent mechanism. J Immunol. 2007;179:2758–65.
52. Johansson SG, Bieber T, Dahl R, Friedmann PS, Lanier BQ, Lockey RF, et al. Revised nomenclature for allergy for global use: report of the Nomenclature Review Committee of the World Allergy Organization, October 2003. J Allergy Clin Immunol. 2004;113(5):832–6.
53. Mustafa SS. Anaphylaxis. In: Kaliner MA, editor. Medscape. http://emedicine.medscape.com/article/135065-overview#showall. Accessed 10 July 2016.
54. Wang J, Sampson HA. Food anaphylaxis. Clin Exp Allergy. 2007;37(5):651–60.
55. Osborne NJ, Koplin JJ, Martin PE, et al. Prevalence of challenge-proven IgE-mediated food allergy using population-based sampling and predetermined challenge criteria in infants. J Allergy Clin Immunol. 2011;127(3):668–76.e1–2.
56. Hourihane JO'B, Kilburn SA, Nordlee JA, Hefle SL, Taylor SL, Warner JO. An evaluation of the sensitivity of subjects with peanut allergy to very low doses of peanut protein: a randomized, double-blind, placebo-controlled food challenge study. J Allergy Clin Immunol. 1997;100(5):596–600.
57. Decker WW, Campbell RL, Manivannan V, et al. The etiology and incidence of anaphylaxis in Rochester, Minnesota: a report from the Rochester Epidemiology Project. J Allergy Clin Immunol. 2008;122(6):1161–5. [Medline]. [Full Text].
58. Greenhawt MJ, Li JT, Bernstein DI, et al. Administering influenza vaccine to egg allergic recipients: a focused practice parameter update. Ann Allergy Asthma Immunol. 2011;106(1):11–6.
59. Centers for Disease Control and Prevention. Prevention and control of influenza with vaccines: recommendations of the Advisory Committee on Immunization Practices (ACIP), 2011. MMWR Morb Mortal Wkly Rep. 2011;60(33):1128–32. [Guideline].
60. Mertes PM, Malinovsky JM, Jouffroy L, et al. Reducing the risk of anaphylaxis during anesthesia: 2011 updated guidelines for clinical practice. J Investig Allergol Clin Immunol. 2011;21(6):442–53.

61. Golden DB. Insect sting anaphylaxis. Immunol Allergy Clin N Am. 2007;27(2):261–72.
62. Gilfillan AM, Tkaczyk C. Integrated signalling pathways for mast-cell activation. Nat Rev Immunol. 2006;6:218–30.
63. Tkaczyk C, Okayama Y, Metcalfe DD, Gilfillan AM. Fcgamma receptors on mast cells: activatory and inhibitory regulation of mediator release. Int Arch Allergy Immunol. 2004;133:305–15.
64. Hong H, Kitaura J, Xiao W, et al. The Src family kinase Hck regulates mast cell activation by suppressing an inhibitory Src family kinase Lyn. Blood. 2007;110:2511–9.
65. Xiao W, Nishimoto H, Hong H, et al. Positive and negative regulation of mast cell activation by Lyn via the FcepsilonRI. J Immunol. 2005;175:6885–92.
66. Parravicini V, Gadina M, Kovarova M, et al. Fyn kinase initiates complementary signals required for IgE-dependent mast cell degranulation. Nat Immunol. 2002;3:741–8.
67. Bansal G, Xie Z, Rao S, et al. Suppression of immunoglobulin E-mediated allergic responses by regulator of G protein signaling 13. Nat Immunol. 2008;9:73–80.

Chapter 4
Risk Factors for Anaphylaxis

4.1 Introduction

It is not possible to predict when anaphylaxis will occur [1, 2]. There is no firm correlation between serum level of immunoglobulin E, how florid the reaction to cutaneous testing has been, or how marked previous reactions were and subsequent anaphylactic response, and this lack of correlation renders accurate prediction impossible [3].

Approaching 20% of children have no skin signs whilst anaphylaxis is occurring [4].

Which organs are involved in anaphylaxis can vary both inter- and intra-individually [3, 5–7] and between episodes.

Having an allergic diathesis increases the risk of anaphylactic reactions. The Rochester Epidemiology Project was able to verify the presence of allergic disease, such as hay fever, asthma, and eczema in 53% of those experiencing anaphylaxis [8]. Thirty-seven percent of those with anaphylaxis in the Memphis study also suffered from other allergic disorders [9]. Other researchers have identified comorbid allergic disorders as a risk for anaphylaxis linked to foodstuffs, radiological contrast media, natural rubber latex, exercise-induced anaphylaxis, and idiopathic anaphylaxis. However, allergic disorders are not linked to higher risk of anaphylaxis following penicillin or insect venom [10].

© Springer Nature Switzerland AG 2020
C. Cingi, N. B. Muluk, *Quick Guide to Anaphylaxis*,
https://doi.org/10.1007/978-3-030-33639-4_4

The route and speed of administering a drug has an effect on the likelihood of anaphylaxis. Giving drugs by mouth is less risky and reactions are typically not as severe although deaths have been recorded in individuals who had eaten foods to which they are allergic. A greater space between exposures lowers the risk that a reaction linked to the production of specific IgE will occur. It is considered likely that breakdown and lesser production of specific IgE over time explains this phenomenon. Where IgE is not involved, such time lags do not have the same effect [10].

A study based in an Accident and Emergency department and which looked at 302 cases of anaphylaxis by review of clinical records identified 87 patients (29% of the sample) with a minimum of one antihypertensive prescribed. This group was at an enhanced risk of symptoms from multiple organ involvement and of being admitted to hospital. The risk of at least three organ systems being involved more than doubled in patients who are taking ACE inhibitors, beta-blockers, diuretics, or indeed antihypertensives generally. The majority of these drugs could also be linked with a greater risk of being admitted to hospital [10–12].

4.2   Factors Affecting the Severity of Reaction

How severe an allergic reaction to food is may be variable, depending on [1, 3]:

- how much of the problem food is swallowed
- the cooked, raw, or processed nature of the food
- which other foods were eaten at the same time

Additional factors affecting severity are [1, 3]:

- The age of the individual
- How sensitised the patient is
- If food is eaten after fasting or swallowed whilst exercising
- The presence or absence of comorbidities such as allergic dermatitis, asthma, or severe hay fever

4.3 Anaphylaxis Risk Factors

Factors affecting the risk of anaphylaxis vary and need to be considered when doctors are presented with cases of anaphylaxis. In a younger case, groundnut allergy increases the risk that the reaction will be extreme. Cases with marked hypersensitivity are at risk from even very small quantities of allergen, and allergen can provoke both extreme and indeed fatal responses. In the case of peanut allergy, an ingested amount measurable in micrograms is sufficient for a reaction [13]. Age additionally compounds risk. Data taken from an anaphylaxis registry indicates that increasing age correlates with increasing relative risk of extreme circulatory symptoms. The age factor odds ratio is 6.06 [14]. During counselling sessions for allergic patients, doctors need to be particularly alert to cardiovascular disorders and make sure that patients with such disorders are under appropriate follow-up. Respiratory disorders have an importance similar to cardiovascular disorders in this respect [15].

A previous anaphylactic reaction is a strong predictor that a subsequent reaction will occur [16–18]. Looking at how severe previous reactions have been appears to be helpful in estimating the subsequent risk of recurrence [19]. Some data point to the fact that a mild reaction in a child may be followed by subsequent more extreme reactions [20]. Being asthmatic appears to confer a high risk of life-threatening anaphylaxis linked to food ingestion [17, 18, 21, 22]. Virtually all cases of anaphylaxis that result in death are linked to asthma [23–25]. However, although asthma is sensitive as a marker of anaphylactic risk, it lacks specificity since asthma is present in approximately one third of food allergy sufferers. In addition, asthma is not a necessary prerequisite for children to have life-threatening anaphylactic reactions. To sum up, whilst having had a previous anaphylactic reaction or comorbid asthma does indeed identify a group within child food allergy sufferers who are at enhanced risk of anaphylaxis, it would appear impossible to identify a group with particularly low risk. Further risk factors involve the quantity and nature of the allergen (groundnut, for instance), where the patient has the reaction, and in which age group they fall (e.g. adolescence). A florid degree of comorbid allergic problems is documented as being linked to greater severity of reaction [19, 24, 25]. All children need to have a comprehensive risk assessment performed which includes all the different factors [14].

A number of studies have indicated that allergic bronchial asthma, if not adequately managed, confers a significant risk of severe anaphylactic reactions [13, 26]. Mastocytosis also confers increased risk [27]. As a result, cases of mastocytosis are advised to have an emergency kit available as a prophylactic measure even should they never have had a marked reaction. The contents of the kit should include an epinephrine auto-injector, steroid, and histamine blocker [15, 28, 29].

We have previously discussed the link between raised tryptase and anaphylaxis linked to insects. Epidemiological research has confirmed that males are at greater risk for developing anaphylactic reactions to insect venom across the entire age range [30]. Up to now, this factor remains unexplained although of interest is the fact that after the age of puberty, boys suffer more illnesses linked to immunoglobulin E than girls, an effect which disappears following puberty [31]. That sex hormones have an influence on how the humoral immune response develops is well known. Drugs similarly can raise the likelihood of an extreme allergic response occurring [15].

Suffers from insect venom allergy are known to have more severe anaphylactic reactions to insect venom if they are taking ACE inhibitors at the time of the reaction. Beta-blockers likely have a similar effect [30]. Other drugs that may work in a similar fashion include aspirin and the NSAIDs. An area currently under investigation is whether these drugs may have the effect of increasing allergen absorption through the gut. Notably, however, certain signalling molecules can have a direct effect on mast cells. It is thought that these mechanisms and others are significant in the pathophysiology [15, 31].

4.4 Patient-Specific Risk Factors

Effects associated with ageing may be responsible for the increasing risk of anaphylaxis with advancing age. Recognition of anaphylaxis may be difficult in infants because they are unable to give a history, whilst some of the signs of anaphylaxis (e.g. skin reddening and hoarseness after crying, regurgitation, or looseness of stools following feeding) may normally observed in healthy infants [32]. Teenaged and young adult patients have a greater likelihood of an anaphylactic reaction triggered by food due to behavioural inconsistency about avoiding known problem foods and unreliability in remembering to carry epinephrine auto-injectors [33]. Whilst anaphylactic reactions are infrequent in pregnant women, those that do occur put both the mother, but especially the unborn child at an elevated risk of death, or irreversible central nervous system damage. Throughout all three trimesters there is a similarity in terms of triggers for anaphylaxis with those in non-pregnant females. Antibiotics of the penicillin group and the other beta-lactams are given prophylactically to prevent infection in infants by group B streptococci at the time of labour and delivery and have thus now become the most frequent triggers for anaphylaxis in pregnancy [34]. Elderly patients run a greater risk of death as a result of anaphylaxis due to various reasons, amongst which are the presence of comorbidity, particularly COPD and circulatory disease, and usage of drugs such as beta-blockers [2, 35–40].

Disorders that may make recognising triggers or the development of symptoms more difficult, for example, visual and hearing deficits, diseases of the neurological system, mental health disorders, autistic spectrum disorder, and delayed development all lead to greater anaphylactic risk [41]. A high degree of hay fever and allergic dermatitis, and even more so, asthma [38], alongside COPD [36] and other disorders of the respiratory system, cardiovascular disorders, [39] and mastocytosis (or any disorder involving a clonal expansion of mast cells [42–45]) are all linked with anaphylactic reactions that are extreme, put life in peril, or actually result in death [2].

Certain drugs taken by patients at the time of an anaphylactic reaction, which include psychopharmacological agents such as diphenhydramine, chlorpheniramine, and first-generation H1 blockers and psychoactive substances, such as alcohol or illicit drugs, may hinder the recognition of anaphylaxis symptoms [37, 41]. A number of drugs used to treat cardiovascular disorders, including beta-blockers and ACE inhibitors, render anaphylaxis treatment more difficult [38–40].

There is also a group of cofactors documented to raise the likelihood of anaphylaxis occurring, but the majority of these have not been studied in a systematic fashion. Co-factors include physical exertion, being exposed to high temperatures or high levels of humidity, disturbed routines, malaise, acute infections such as those affecting the upper respiratory tract, psychological stress, menstruation (premenstrual and ovulatory stages), and having taken alcohol or aspirin and other NSAIDs [2, 37, 41, 46–48].

4.4.1   Risk Assessment in Anaphylaxis [2, 37]

Factors known to increase the likelihood of anaphylaxis, whether or not it results in death, are the following:

1. Age. During adolescence and young adulthood there is an elevated risk of dying from anaphylaxis related to food allergy. In old age, anaphylactic reactions to insect venom are more deadly.
2. Comorbid disorders:
   - asthma
   - circulatory disorders
   - mental health disorders (acting by hindering symptomatic recognition)
   - mastocytosis (whether symptoms are apparent or not)
   - mutations of the KIT gene that result in activation

- thyroid disorders (for a subset of cases of idiopathic anaphylaxis)
- decreased activity by the platelet-activating factor acetyl-hydrolase enzyme
- allergic disorders characterised by high levels of histamine in the blood, and occurring through IgE mechanisms
- psychological stress
- acute infection
- diminished host-defensive capability

3. Use of substances (medicinal or recreational) at the time of the episode:

- substances which may make it more difficult to recognise anaphylactic symptoms, such as alcohol, illicit drugs, sedating drugs, and hypnotics
- substances that make anaphylaxis more severe, such as beta-blockers, ACE inhibitors, and angiotensin II receptor antagonists

4. Other factors of relevance include how severe prior episodes of anaphylaxis have been, and whether they have primed future responses, a high level of physical exertion, and certain occupations.

5. Allergens intrinsically more capable of provoking anaphylaxis:

- foods include groundnuts, tree nuts, fish that possess fins, shellfish, eggs, dairy products, and sesame
- insect stings or bites. Of particular importance are the stinging Hymenopterids (bee, wasp, and ant families) and biting insects such as mosquitoes, kissing bugs, and pigeon ticks
- inhaled allergens such as dander from cats, hamsters, and horses, or grass pollen
- latex rubber
- drugs, in particular the beta-lactams and agents used for neuromuscular blockade.

References

1. Boyce JA, Assa'ad A, Burks AW, et al. Guidelines for the diagnosis and management of food allergy in the United States: report of the NIAID-sponsored expert panel. J Allergy Clin Immunol. 2010;126(6 Suppl):S1–S58.
2. Simons FE. Anaphylaxis: recent advances in assessment and treatment. J Allergy Clin Immunol. 2009;124(4):625–36.
3. Anaphylaxis risk factors. https://www.epipen.com/en/hcp/about-anaphylaxis/anaphylaxis-risk-factors. Accessed 11 July 2016.
4. Järvinen KM, Celestin J. Anaphylaxis avoidance and management: educating patients and their caregivers. J Asthma Allergy. 2014;7:95–104.
5. Dinakar C. Anaphylaxis in children: current understanding and key issues in diagnosis and treatment. Curr Allergy Asthma Rep. 2012;12(6):641–9.
6. Lieberman P, Nicklas RA, Oppenheimer J, et al. The diagnosis and management of anaphylaxis practice parameter: 2010 update. J Allergy Clin Immunol. 2010;126(3):477–80.e1–42.
7. Simons FE. Anaphylaxis. J Allergy Clin Immunol. 2010;125(2 Suppl 2):S161–81.
8. Decker WW, Campbell RL, Manivannan V, et al. The etiology and incidence of anaphylaxis in Rochester, Minnesota: a report from the Rochester Epidemiology Project. J Allergy Clin Immunol. 2008;122(6):1161–5.
9. Webb LM, Lieberman P. Anaphylaxis: a review of 601 cases. Ann Allergy Asthma Immunol. 2006;97(1):39–43.
10. Mustafa SS. Anaphylaxis. In: Kaliner MA, editor. Medscape. http://emedicine.medscape.com/article/135065-overview#showall.
11. Boggs W. Anaphylaxis worse with antihypertensive medication. Medscape Medical News. 2013. http://www.medscape.com/viewarticle/781274. Accessed April 2, 2013.
12. Lee S, Hess EP, Nestler DM, Bellamkonda Athmaram VR, Bellolio MF, Decker WW, et al. Antihypertensive medication use is associated with increased organ system involvement and hospitalization in emergency department patients with anaphylaxis. J Allergy Clin Immunol. 2013;131(4):1103–8.
13. Sicherer SH, Sampson HA. Peanut allergy: emerging concepts and approaches for an apparent epidemic. J Allergy Clin Immunol. 2007;120:491–503; quiz 504–5.
14. Muraro A, Roberts G, Clark A, Eigenmann PA, Halken S, Lack G, Moneret-Vautrin A, Niggemann B, Rancé F, EAACI Task Force on Anaphylaxis in Children. The management of anaphylaxis in

childhood: position paper of the European academy of allergology andclinical immunology. Allergy. 2007;62(8):857–71. Epub 2007 Jun 21.

15. Worm M, Babina M, Hompes S. Causes and risk factors for anaphylaxis. J Dtsch Dermatol Ges. 2013;11(1):44–50. https://doi.org/10.1111/j.1610-0387.2012.08045.x. Epub 2012 Nov 26.

16. Lantner R, Reisman RE. Clinical and immunologic features and subsequent course of patients with severe insectsting anaphylaxis. J Allergy Clin Immunol. 1989;84:900–6.

17. Mullins RJ. Anaphylaxis: risk factors for recurrence. Clin Exp Allergy. 2003;33:1033–40.

18. Pumphrey RS, Stanworth SJ. The clinical spectrum of anaphylaxis in northwest England. Clin Exp Allergy. 1996;26:1364–70.

19. Hourihane JO, Grimshaw KE, Lewis SA, Briggs RA, Trewin JB, King RM, et al. Does severity of low-dose, doubleblind, placebo-controlled, food challenge reflect severity of allergic reactions to peanut in the community. Clin Exp Allergy. 2005;35:1227–33.

20. Vander Leek TK, Liu AH, Stefanski K, Blacker B, Bock SA. The natural history of peanut allergy in young children and its association with serum peanutspecific IgE. J Pediatr. 2000;137:749–55.

21. Sampson HA. Anaphylaxis and emergency treatment. Pediatrics. 2003;111S:1601–7.

22. Sampson HA. Fatal food-induced anaphylaxis. Allergy. 1998;53(Suppl. 46):125–30.

23. Pumphrey RS. Lessons for management of anaphylaxis from a study of fatal reactions. Clin Exp Allergy. 2000;30:1144–50.

24. Sampson HA, Mendelson L, Rosen JP. Fatal and near-fatal anaphylactic reactions to food in children and adolescents. N Engl J Med. 1992;327:380–4.

25. Pumphrey R. Anaphylaxis: can we tell who is at risk of a fatal reaction? Curr Opin Allergy Clin Immunol. 2004;4:285–90.

26. Iribarren C, Tolstykh IV, Miller MK, Eisner MD. Asthma and the prospective risk of anaphylactic shock and other allergy diagnoses in a large integrated health care delivery system. Ann Allergy Asthma Immunol. 2010;104:371–7.

27. Brockow K, Ring J. Update on diagnosis and treatment of mastocytosis. Curr Allergy Asthma Rep. 2011;11:292–9.

28. Simons KJ, Simons FE. Epinephrine and its use in anaphylaxis: current issues. Curr Opin Allergy Clin Immunol. 2010;10:354–61.

29. Ring J, Brockow K, Duda D, Eschenhagen T, Fuchs T, Hutteger I, Kapp A, Klimek L, Müller U, Niggemann B, Pfaar O, Przybilla B, Rebien W, Rietschel E, Ruëff F, Schnadt S, Tryba M, Worm M, Sitter H, Schultze-Werninghaus G. Akuttherapie anaphylaktischer Reaktionen. Allergo J. 2007;16:420–34.

30. Ruëff F, Przybilla B, Bilo MB, Müller U, Scheipl F, Aberer W, Birnbaum J, Bodzenta-Lukaszyk A, Bonifazi F, Bucher C, Campi P, Darsow U, Egger C, Haeberli G, Hawranek T, Körner M, Kucharewicz I, Kuchenhoff H, Lang R, Quercia O, Reider N, Severino M, Sticherling M, Sturm GJ, Wüthrich B. Predictors of severe systemic anaphylactic reactions in patients with Hymenoptera venom allergy: importance of baseline serum tryptase—a study of the European Academy of Allergology and Clinical Immunology Interest Group on Insect Venom Hypersensitivity. J Allergy Clin Immunol. 2009;124:1047–54.
31. Chen W, Mempel M, Schober W, Behrendt H, Ring J. Gender difference, sex hormones, and immediate type hypersensitivity reactions. Allergy. 2008;63:1418–27.
32. Simons FER. Anaphylaxis in infants: can recognition and management be improved? J Allergy Clin Immunol. 2007;120:537–40.
33. Greenhawt MJ, Singer AM, Baptist AP. Food allergy and food allergy attitudes among college students. J Allergy Clin Immunol. 2009;124:323–7.
34. Chaudhuri K, Gonzales J, Jesurun CA, Ambat MT, Mandal-Chaudhuri S. Anaphylactic shock in pregnancy: a case study and review of the literature. Int J Obstet Anesth. 2008;17:350–7.
35. Lieberman PL. Anaphylaxis. In: Adkinson Jr NF, Bochner BS, Busse WW, Holgate ST, Lemanske Jr RF, Simons FER, editors. Middleton's allergy: principles and practice. 7th ed. St. Louis: Mosby; 2009. p. 1027–49.
36. Greenberger PA, Rotskoff BD, Lifschultz B. Fatal anaphylaxis: postmortem findings and associated comorbid diseases. Ann Allergy Asthma Immunol. 2007;98:252–7.
37. Simons FER, Frew AJ, Ansotegui IJ, Bochner BS, Finkelman F, Golden DBK, et al. Risk assessment in anaphylaxis: current and future approaches. J Allergy Clin Immunol. 2007;120(suppl):S2–S24.
38. Summers CW, Pumphrey RS, Woods CN, McDowell G, Pemberton PW, Arkwright PD. Factors predicting anaphylaxis to peanuts and tree nuts in patients referred to a specialist center. J Allergy Clin Immunol. 2008;121:632–8.
39. Mueller UR. Cardiovascular disease and anaphylaxis. Curr Opin Allergy Clin Immunol. 2007;7:337–41.
40. Lang DM. Do beta-blockers really enhance the risk of anaphylaxis during immunotherapy? Curr Allergy Asthma Rep. 2008;8:37–44.
41. Simons FER. Anaphylaxis, killer allergy: long-term management in the community. J Allergy Clin Immunol. 2006;117:367–77.
42. Gonzalez de Olano D, de la Hoz Caballer B, Nunez Lopez R, Sanchez-Munoz L, Cuevas Agustin M, Dieguez MC, et al. Prevalence of allergy and anaphylactic symptoms in 210 adult

and pediatric patients with mastocytosis in Spain: a study of the Spanish network on mastocytosis (REMA). Clin Exp Allergy. 2007;37:1547–55.

43. Brockow K, Jofer C, Behrendt H, Ring J. Anaphylaxis in patients with mastocytosis: a study on history, clinical features and risk factors in 120 patients. Allergy. 2008;63:226–32.

44. Bonadonna P, Perbellini O, Passalacqua G, Caruso B, Colarossi S, Dal Fior D, et al. Clonal mast cell disorders in patients with systemic reactions to Hymenoptera stings and increased serum tryptase levels. J Allergy Clin Immunol. 2009;123:680–6.

45. Muller UR. Elevated baseline serum tryptase, mastocytosis and anaphylaxis. Clin Exp Allergy. 2009;39:620–2.

46. Pumphrey RSH, Gowland MH. Further fatal allergic reactions to food in the United Kingdom, 1999-2006. J Allergy Clin Immunol. 2007;119:1018–9.

47. Du Toit G. Food-dependent exercise-induced anaphylaxis in childhood. Pediatr Allergy Immunol. 2007;18:455–63.

48. Fernando SL. Cold-induced anaphylaxis. J Pediatr. 2009;154:148.

Chapter 5
Symptoms and Findings for Anaphylaxis

5.1 Introduction

Anaphylaxis involves multiple organ systems and is intense in severity. The most readily observable signs occur within the skin, respiratory, cardiovascular and respiratory systems, and the gut. Much research has focused on the symptomatology and signs as grouped by organ system. It is frequent to observe mucocutaneous and cutaneous manifestations of anaphylaxis. In greater than 90% of cases, the signs consist of a mixture of hives, erythema, itching, and angioedema. To takes an example, the Memphis study [1] reported that hives and/or angioedema was seen in 87% of instances of anaphylaxis. The rates of mucocutaneous involvement as reported elsewhere are similar [2].

There is typically involvement of the upper airway, with blockage of the nose, sternutation, and signs resembling a cold. Coughing, a change in vocal quality, or feeling constricted in the throat area may presage the development of severe airway compromise. This may be accompanied by conjunctival injection. Spasm of the bronchi or swelling of the upper airway may provoke dyspnoea. The resultant fall in blood pressure and oxygenation may result in fainting, lightheadedness, or loss of consciousness. Bronchospasm or ischaemic myocardium may produce pain in the chest. Whilst gut manifestations (vomiting,

© Springer Nature Switzerland AG 2020
C. Cingi, N. B. Muluk, *Quick Guide to Anaphylaxis*,
https://doi.org/10.1007/978-3-030-33639-4_5

nausea, diarrhoea) also occur, they are less fundamental than other signs, except in cases of food allergy. In the Memphis study, the rates for dyspnoea, fainting, and diarrhoea/griping were 59%, 33%, and 29%, respectively [1].

Anaphylactic responses most frequently involve the skin, respiratory and cardiovascular systems, and the gut. Between 80 and 90% of anaphylaxis involves the skin and mucosal surfaces of the body. The majority of adult cases are characterised by a mixture of hives, itching, redness, and angioedema. Despite this, young cases may show respiratory signs without skin involvement, but why this should be so is unknown [3]. It must be added, too, that the gravest types of anaphylaxis happen with no cutaneous manifestations [2].

Anaphylaxis may present as loss of consciousness. It is common for patients to complain of angor animi. Whilst anaphylaxis may present with symptoms confined to a single organ system, typically, a minimum of two organ systems are involved, as would be expected in what is essentially a systemic problem [4].

Initial presentations characteristically involve itching and erythema. Alongside these manifestations, a constellation of other symptoms may rapidly develop, such as [2, 4]:

- Cutaneous (visible) signs: flushed appearance, hives, erythema with or without conjunctival injection, itching, feeling hot, oedema, widespread redness, swelling around the eyes, lacrimation.
- Respiratory: lingual, oropharyngeal, or laryngeal angioedema may obstruct the upper airway. There may be bronchospasm, chest tightness, dyspnoea, nasal congestion, running nose, throat constriction, audible wheeze, and coughing.
- Oral: itching around the mouth, altered taste sensation, labiolingual swelling.
- Cardiovascular: lightheadedness, malaise, fainting, central chest pain, palpitations, low blood pressure, rhythm alterations, and circulatory shock.

- Gut-related: difficulty swallowing, nausea and vomiting, diarrhoea, griping, abdominodynia, excessive gut motility leading to faecal incontinence.
- Central nervous system: headache, vertigo, blurring of vision, and, very rarely, convulsions.
- Urinary urgency and incontinence of urine.
- Other: metallic taste, angor animi.

The initial presenting symptoms develop rapidly and reach a climax 3–30 min after first onset. On occasion, a latency period of between 1 and 8 h may intervene, in which case the anaphylactic response is termed biphasic. A prolonged variant may occur with symptoms lasting a significant length of time. Death may occur within minutes of the onset of symptoms, although, in rare cases, a death may occur days or weeks after the initial response [4].

Anaphylactic responses may be idiosyncratic, such that a mildly allergic response may become life-threatening in severity when the antigen is re-encountered. As an example, a nut allergy sufferer who accidentally consumes a nut might experience only slight swelling periorally and tearing on one occasion, but when re-exposure occurs, there may be a full-blown reaction with a potentially fatal outcome, characterised by dyspnoea, vertigo, urticaria, and impalpable pulse. Whilst both scenarios represent anaphylaxis, there is little overlap between the presentations in terms of symptomatology or probable outcome [5].

Circulatory shock is one amongst several potential consequences of anaphylaxis. It is secondary to hypoperfusion of the organ capillary beds during anaphylaxis. However, shock is by no means an invariable concomitant to anaphylaxis. A study conducted over a decade found no shock in the anaphylaxis cases considered. Thus, "anaphylaxis" and "anaphylactic shock" are not interchangeable terms. Anaphylaxis is a broader term which also encompasses anaphylactic shock [5].

5.2   Physical Examination

The key element in the physical examination is establishing whether the airway is patent, assessing respiratory rate and evaluating the level of consciousness (e.g. alertness, orientation, and coherence).

General findings depend on how severe the anaphylaxis has become and which organ system is primarily affected. Vital signs may be abnormal, with tachycardia, elevated respiratory rate plus/minus hypotension [2].

Patients are often disturbed by intense itching. Large-scale catecholamine release results in anxiety, shaking, and feeling cold. Usually, a patient will have a sense of foreboding except where conscious level is impaired by hypotension or hypoxia. In extreme cases, circulatory collapse and respiratory arrest may supervene [2].

5.2.1   Respiratory Findings

Severe labiolingual angioedema (as may occur on occasion with ACE inhibitors) may block the airway. Swelling of the larynx may manifest as stridor or aerophagia. Dysphonia, hoarseness, or losing one's voice are all possible signs. Wheezing may be secondary to spasm of the bronchi, swollen airways, and excessive mucous secretion. During an operation, bronchospasm may be noticed as increased ventilatory pressure. Total occlusion of the airway is recognised as the principal cause of anaphylactic mortalities [2].

5.2.2   Cardiovascular Findings

In a quarter of cases, tachycardia occurs, mostly secondary to hypovolaemia and catecholamine release. Bradycardic response, in contrast, usually reflects vasovagally mediated vasodepression. Whilst tachycardia is more typically noted, bradycardia may also occur. Thus, the presence of bradycardia may be less useful diagnostically than was once thought. A relative slowing of the heart in the context of low perfusion pressure has been observed in experimental settings involving insect venom anaphylaxis, and in addition, has been seen in trauma cases [6–10].

Loss of consciousness may be due to hypotension, itself the result of massive vasodilation, and hypoxic myocardial damage. Cardiovascular collapse and circulatory shock may be the only presenting features, an important factor to consider in perioperative and intraoperative settings. Given that shock may present without evidence of cutaneous change, anaphylaxis must be included in the differential diagnosis for cases with no identifiable trigger [2].

5.2.3 Cognitive Findings

Obtunded consciousness, which may present as either disorientation or aggression, can be the result of hypoperfusion +/− hypoxia.

5.2.4 Cutaneous Findings

The most significant clinical sign is urticaria. Hives may be seen at any anatomical location, but are especially prevalent on areas where the dermal thickness is less, such as the palms and soles, or the medial aspect of the thighs. The hives are red and raised, with blanched areas visible on occasion. They produce marked pruritus. The border varies and they may be of several different sizes. If two or more lesions coalesce, giant urticaria results. Sometimes the entire skin may be erythematous and oedematous [2].

By contrast with a systemic reaction, such as that happens in anaphylaxis, a localised allergic response, e.g. to insect venom, is restricted to one area, has surrounding erythema and produces pruritus, but will be unlikely to cause respiratory difficulty. If a lesion is localised, then, despite the severity of the lesion, it does not point towards anaphylaxis occurring [2].

Angioedema (a friable area of oedema) is also often seen and involves deeper strata of the dermis. It does not pit, nor produce itching. The main areas where it may be observed are the throat, perioral region, blephara, hands and feet, and genitalia. A systemic erythematous response lacking hives or angioedema may also be seen on occasion. Skin manifestations may appear late or not at all if anaphylaxis progresses quickly [2].

5.2.5   Gastrointestinal Findings

Vomiting, diarrhoea, and bloating of the abdomen are often noted [2].

5.3   Clinical Presentation

5.3.1   Clinical Manifestations of Anaphylaxis

From a clinical viewpoint, anaphylaxis presents as a generalised disorder of a severe kind, affecting the respiratory and circulatory systems and producing symptoms such as stridor, wheeze, and low blood pressure. Left untreated, it may worsen and lead to death. If IgE mediates the response, the signs appear within 2 h of exposure to the antigen. Allergic anaphylactic responses to food usually happen within 30 min of ingestion, but even more quickly if intravenous drugs or insect venoms are the culprits. In the bulk of cases, skin signs are present, even more so in younger people [3, 11–13].

Whilst itching palms, feet, or head may presage the development of anaphylaxis, it is important to be aware that anaphylaxis may occur in the absence of any signs in the skin. For children, the most worrying development is bronchospasm [3, 12, 14, 15]. Where there are any signs that the airway is affected (such as swelling of the larynx, stridor, difficulty speaking, becoming mute, and experiencing dyspnoea), doctors need to be alert to the gravity of the problem. It is less common to find circulatory compromise as an early sign in teenagers [3, 15]. Alongside hypotension, patients may feel dizzy, have angor animi, and obtunded consciousness level. Severe griping, with possible heaving and loose stools, may herald the onset of severe anaphylaxis [11]. Other initial signs may be a marked nasal discharge, and periocular and nasal pruritus, that begins abruptly. Using a grading scale can be beneficial, and helps guide the appropriate use of epinephrine [16]. A study looking at hospitalised children in the USA with anaphylaxis [15] reported a rate of 6% for biphasic or discontinuous episodes, and 3% were severe in intensity. Ninety percent of intermittent type anaphylaxis occurred within 4–12 h of the main attack. If epinephrine is not promptly administered, the likelihood of biphasic anaphylaxis increases [17–20]. Some patients also have a persistent type response that lasts for hours. Exercise-induced anaphylaxis (EIA) features hives, upper airway restriction, and circulatory collapse [21, 22]. It only occurs following exercise. This is a disorder mostly affecting younger patients, and on many occasions is linked to food (i.e. food-dependent EIA) [13].

5.4 Complications

It is rare for patients to suffer complications from anaphylaxis, and recovery is usually complete. Hypoxia and hypotension may lead to ischaemia of the myocardium, especially if there coexists asymptomatic coronary arteriosclerosis. Administering agents to raise the blood pressure may actually provoke ischaemia or rhythm disorders. Cerebral damage can be caused by hypoxia if it is prolonged. Occasionally, anaphylaxis resulting in syncope may lead to injury through falling. If bronchospasm or swelling of the larynx are sufficient to cause respiratory arrest, hypoxic cerebral injury can result [2].

References

1. Webb LM, Lieberman P. Anaphylaxis: a review of 601 cases. Ann Allergy Asthma Immunol. 2006;97(1):39–43.
2. Mustafa SS. Anaphylaxis. In: Kaliner MA, editor. Medscape. http://emedicine.medscape.com/article/135065-overview#showall. Accessed 11 July 2016.
3. Braganza SC, Acworth JP, Mckinnon DR, Peake JE, Brown AF. Paediatric emergency department anaphylaxis: different patterns from adults. Arch Dis Child. 2006;91(2):159–63.
4. Lockey RF. Anaphylaxis: synopsis. http://www.worldallergy.org/professional/allergic_diseases_center/anaphylaxis/anaphylaxis-synopsis.php. Accessed 11 July 2016.
5. Anaphylaxis Symptoms. EpiPen. https://www.epipen.com/what-is-anaphylaxis/anaphylaxis-symptoms. Accessed 11 July 2016.
6. Schadt JC, Ludbrook J. Hemodynamic and neurohumoral responses to acute hypovolemia in conscious mammals. Am J Phys. 1991;260(2 Pt 2):H305–18.
7. Demetriades D, Chan LS, Bhasin P, Berne TV, Ramicone E, Huicochea F, et al. Relative bradycardia in patients with traumatic hypotension. J Trauma. 1998;45(3):534–9.
8. Smith PL, Kagey-Sobotka A, Bleecker ER, et al. Physiologic manifestations of human anaphylaxis. J Clin Invest. 1980;66(5):1072–80.
9. van der Linden PW, Struyvenberg A, Kraaijenhagen RJ, Hack CE, van der Zwan JK. Anaphylactic shock after insect-sting challenge in 138 persons with a previous insect-sting reaction. Ann Intern Med. 1993;118(3):161–8.
10. Brown SG, Blackman KE, Stenlake V, Heddle RJ. Insect sting anaphylaxis; prospective evaluation of treatment with intravenous adrenaline and volume resuscitation. Emerg Med J. 2004;21(2):149–54.
11. Brown SGA. Clinical features and severity grading of anaphylaxis. J Allergy Clin Immunol. 2004;114:371–6.
12. Bohlke K, Davis RL, De Stefano F, Mary SM, Braun MM, Thompson RS. Epidemiology of anaphylaxis among children and adolescents enrolled in a health maintenance organization. J Allergy Clin Immunol. 2004;113:536–42.
13. Muraro A, Roberts G, Clark A, Eigenmann PA, Halken S, Lack G, Moneret-Vautrin A, Niggemann B, Rancé F, EAACI Task Force on Anaphylaxis in Children. The management of anaphylaxis in childhood: position paper of the European academy of allergology andclinical immunology. Allergy. 2007;62(8):857–71. Epub 2007 Jun 21.

14. Sampson HA, Mendelson L, Rosen JP. Fatal and near-fatal ana-
    phylactic reactions to food in children and adolescents. N Engl J
    Med. 1992;327:380–4.
15. Dibs S, Baker M. Anaphylaxis in children: a 5-year experience.
    Pediatrics. 1997;99:1–5.
16. Sampson HA. Anaphylaxis and emergency treatment. Pediatrics.
    2003;111S:1601–7.
17. Lee JM, Greenes DS. Biphasic anaphylactic reactions in pediat-
    rics. Pediatrics. 2000;106:762–6.
18. Sampson HA. Fatal food-induced anaphylaxis. Allergy.
    1998;53(Suppl. 46):125–30.
19. Lieberman P. Biphasic anaphylactic reactions. Ann Allergy
    Asthma Immunol. 2005;95:217–26.
20. Ellis AK, Day JH. Incidence and characteristics of biphasic ana-
    phylaxis: a prospective evaluation of 103 patients. Ann Allergy
    Asthma Immunol. 2007;98:64–9.
21. Romano A, Di Fonso M, Giuffreda F, Papa G, Artesani MC, Viola
    M, et al. Food-dependent exercise-induced anaphylaxis: clinical
    and laboratory findings in 54 subjects. Int Arch Allergy Immunol.
    2001;125:264–72.
22. Tewari A, Du Toit G, Lack G. The difficulties of diagnosing food-
    dependent exercise-induced anaphylaxis in childhood—a case
    study and review. Pediatr Allergy Immunol. 2006;17:157–60.

Chapter 6
Diagnosis and Laboratory Tests for Anaphylaxis

6.1 Diagnosis

The diagnosis of anaphylaxis is clinical. Physical examination should primarily focus on the patency of the airway, respiratory rate, perfusion, and exclude obtundation of consciousness (by checking orientation, alertness, and coherence) [1].

The following physical signs may be expected to occur [1]:

- Overall appearance and vital signs differ depending on the severity of the anaphylaxis and which organs are involved. Typically, a sufferer will be distressed and agitated.
- Respiratory signs include marked lingual and labial angioedema, raised respiratory rate, stridor and severe urge to breathe deeply, losing one's voice, dysphonia +/− change in quality of voice. Sufferers often wheeze.
- Circulatory system signs include being tachycardic and hypotensive. Cardiovascular collapse and circulatory shock may rapidly intervene. This may be the sole finding.
- Central nervous system involvement is apparent through obtundation of consciousness, disorientation, and aggressive or agitated behaviour.
- Cutaneous signs may include the archetypal urticarial reaction (hive formation) at any body site, angioedematous

© Springer Nature Switzerland AG 2020
C. Cingi, N. B. Muluk, *Quick Guide to Anaphylaxis*,
https://doi.org/10.1007/978-3-030-33639-4_6

swelling of soft tissues, or flushing or confluent erythematous rash alone, without other cutaneous signs.
- Gut symptoms include vomiting, loose stools, and a distended abdomen.

To diagnose anaphylaxis, it is necessary to have a clinical suspicion and to recognise that the risk exists. If at least one of the following three groups of signs occurs over the space of a few minutes or hours, anaphylaxis is likely [1]:

- Acute phase signs of cutaneous +/− mucosal surfaces, plus at least one of the following: respiratory alterations, hypotension, and failure of end organs.
- At least two of the following occur rapidly following exposure to a suspected allergen: hypotension, respiratory difficulty, gut symptoms that persist, or skin or mucosal changes.
- Hypotensive episode, not considered a simple side effect, after exposure to a previously known allergen, inappropriately low BP or a systolic value less than 30% of the normal expected value.

In fact, anaphylaxis runs the full spectrum from seemingly mild initial presentation through to a situation where circulatory of respiratory collapse can occur. It is highly dangerous to delay diagnosis of anaphylaxis until a point where systemic involvement is certain. At the onset of clinical signs of anaphylaxis, it is very challenging to predict with any accuracy how the subsequent syndrome will develop [1].

Some important differential diagnoses to bear in mind when anaphylaxis is suspected include the following [1]:

- Vasovagal episode causing decreased vasomotor tone (probably the most common mimic of anaphylaxis)
- *Globus hystericus*
- Hereditary angioedema
- Other causes of shock (specifically, hypovolaemic, cardiogenic, or septic)
- Disorders that produce a flushing response, such as Red Man Syndrome with vancomycin, pancreatic polypeptide-secreting

neoplasms, menopause, response to alcohol consumption, and epilepsy producing autonomic signs
- Monosodium glutamate intolerance
- Scombroid fish poisoning
- Clarkson's syndrome
- Pulmonary embolism
- Myocardial infarction
- Foreign body lodged in an airway (suspect in younger children)
- Poisoning, acute
- Neurological origin (cerebrovascular accident, convulsion)
- Psychogenic cause, such as panic attack, overbreathing. Vocal cord dysfunction syndrome or somatoform anaphylaxis

6.2 Laboratory Testing

Mast cells and basophils are central actors in the development of a systemic anaphylactic response. Both release and production of chemical mediators by these cell types account for the majority of the features of a systemic anaphylactic response. The two most well-studied and understood amongst the various mediators are tryptase and histamine. On occasion, increased circulating tryptase and histamine levels may be seen in venous samples taken when symptoms are just beginning. Furthermore, histamine, histaminic metabolites (N-methylhistamine and N-methylimidazole ethanoic acid), and 11-beta-PGF2-alpha (11β-PGF2α), metabolised from prostaglandin (PG) D2 metabolite, may be quantified in urine following an episode of anaphylaxis [2].

Specialist laboratory investigations are not usually necessary, but may occasionally prove of benefit. Nonetheless, where confusion about the diagnosis exists (as may occur with intermittent occurrence), or a differential diagnosis warrants exclusion, the following specialist investigations may on occasion be contemplated [2]:

- Tryptase (blood level)
- Histamine (blood level)
- Levels of histaminic metabolites (N-methylhistamine and *N*-methylimidazole ethanoic acid) and 11-beta-PGF2-alpha (11β-PGF2α), metabolised from prostaglandin (PG) D2, may be available from specific private laboratories [2].

Chymase and mast cell carboxypeptidase A3 are similarly used in the diagnosis of anaphylaxis, despite their needing further investigation in terms of biomarker status, and the lack of reference intervals for routine use [3].

Serum tryptase specimens should be taken between 15 min and 3 h of the start of an anaphylactic reaction. Ideally, the level would be compared with baseline evaluation, or, in the worst case scenario, with a level taken 24 h after the complete cessation of clinical features of anaphylaxis. Levels measured during research into insect venom anaphylaxis demonstrated a peak in blood tryptase between 15 min and 1 h after initial anaphylactic onset, and fall thereafter, with tryptase having a half-life of approximately 2 h [4, 5]. A high initial peak in tryptase level may still leave traces for several hours after the episode [2].

The peak seen in histamine levels is even more transitory. Blood levels are at their maximum within 5–10 min of anaphylactic onset, but the short half-life (1–2 min) means that levels return to baseline within 15–30 min [4, 6–8]. As a result, blood samples should be taken as soon as possible, and, wherever practical, no more than 30 min after initial signs appear. The serum levels of histaminic metabolites have a slightly longer half-life, and urinary samples may reveal their presence for a considerable period [2].

To identify the trigger for the episode, skin prick tests or laboratory IgE serology may be of value. An investigation may incorporate tests for the following:

- Single or multiple food allergies
- Drug allergy
- Non-IgE-mediated hypersensitivity responses

6.2.1 Histamine and Tryptase Assessment

If a patient happens to present in the immediate aftermath of an anaphylactic attack, taking blood levels of histamine and its metabolites in urine, or blood levels of tryptase, may be of value in confirming anaphylaxis has occurred [9].

Circulating histamine levels rise within 10 min of the onset of anaphylaxis, but drop again within 30 min. In general, urinary histamine determinations are plagued by the complex effects of diet and the urinary microbial flora. Determining histaminic metabolites in the urine is more advisable, but such tests are typically not easily accessed by clinicians [1].

Levels of beta-tryptase (aka mature tryptase) peak within one and a half hours after initial onset of the attack and may be persistent for anything up to 5 h. A study examining 259 cases of anaphylaxis related to anaesthesia found a positive predictive rate of raised tryptase of 92.6%, whilst the negative predictive rate of a normal tryptase level was 54.3%. It is possible that taking a series of levels may improve the predictive value, but further research is needed to clarify the picture [1].

Checking the baseline tryptase level between episodes of anaphylaxis can help to exclude systemic mastocytosis as a differential diagnosis. Cases of mastocytosis are associated with significantly raised levels of alpha-tryptase, but in unaffected individuals, serum alpha-tryptase should be normal. In a case of suspected anaphylaxis, a combined tryptase level (alpha- and beta-tryptase) of 20 or above points towards mastocytosis, whilst a level below 10 points away from mastocytosis as diagnosis [1].

Recent research into anaphylaxis occurring as a result of insect venom allergy emphasises that detailed examination of tryptase level may be appropriate, especially in cases characterised by hypotension [10–12]. If the baseline value for tryptase is above 11.4 μg/L, the differential diagnosis should include both mastocytosis and a monoclonal proliferative lesion (e.g. c-pack mutation) and workup may need bone marrow trephine and cytogenetics [11, 12].

Ascertaining a rise in either histamine or tryptase can prove challenging, and in some cases only one of these parameters may be elevated. A study looking at 97 patients attending Accident and Emergency for severe allergic reactions found that 42 cases had an elevated histamine, whilst 20 had elevated tryptamine [13]. There was no correlation between a rise in one marker and a change in the other [1].

Candidate biomarkers are currently under investigation, including platelet-activating factor (PAF), bradykinin, chymase, mast cell carboxypeptidase A3, dipeptidyl peptidase I, IL-33 and a number of other cytokines, leukotrienes, and prostaglandins [14]. In cases where anaphylaxis has proven fatal, PAF acetylhydrolase levels have been found to be low, and it is conceivable that severe or fatal cases are caused by a failure to inactivate PAF. Thus, the enzyme may have a role as a biomarker [3].

6.2.1.1   Tryptase

Mast cells and basophils jointly produce tryptase, but mast cells contain 500 times greater levels than basophils [15–17]. Mast cells undergo degranulation when activated, resulting in secretion of both tryptase and histamine. Given that tryptase typically originates from mast cells predominantly, elevated tryptase levels usually indicate mast cell involvement [18]. The molecular biology of tryptase is still awaiting complete characterisation, but is known to exist in both a mature and proform [2]:

- The proform (protryptase) undergoes acute release into blood by mast cells when unactivated [19]. It is unknown what role protryptase plays physiologically, other than as the substrate for conversion into beta-tryptase [20]. Conversion takes the form of proteolysis [21].
- Beta-tryptase is stored in secretory granules within the mast cell cytoplasm as a tetrameric enzyme [22], complexed with heparin proteoglycan [23, 24]. When mast cells are stimulated, both mature tryptase and histamine are released extra-

cellularly. Laboratory studies show that tryptase initiates anaphylatoxin release, causes the inactivation of fibrinogen, and stimulates a number of different cell lineages. However, its role in vivo has still not been fully determined. Unlike beta-tryptase, alpha-tryptase exhibits minimal protease actions [2].

The genes for the principal tryptases in man are located on chromosome 16. The TPSAB1 gene contains information to produce both alpha and beta-tryptases, whilst TPSB2 encodes only beta-tryptase without further modification. Humans possess 4 alleles for the tryptase gene, two of which come from each parent. In approximately 25% of individuals, there are two alpha and two beta alleles, around 50% have one alpha and three beta alleles, and the remaining 25% have four beta alleles [2].

Normally, unless an individual has had an anaphylactic attack within the preceding 4 h, tryptase is undetectable in adult blood since its level is below 1 ng/mL. A baseline value of 1–11.4 ng/mL is found, with a reference range of 3–5 ng/mL. Healthy women have a level approximately 0.2 ng/mL higher than that found in healthy men.

A raised level of all forms of tryptase or beta-tryptase only may have a diagnostic utility in differentiating anaphylaxis from conditions that mimic the symptoms, such as a vasovagal attack, sepsis, convulsion, myocardial infarction, flushing, or carcinoid tumours. In such cases, tryptase as a whole or as beta-tryptase is not elevated [2].

A raised beta-tryptase blood level indicates mast cell activation (plus, possibly, basophil activation). No other conditions are known which give similar peaks in tryptase. Total tryptase may also rise to a peak in anaphylaxis, such that total tryptase level has the same sensitivity as beta-tryptase alone [25]. A total tryptase that exceeds $2 + (1.2 \times \text{baseline value})$ is clinically significant [26]. In systemic anaphylactic responses, total tryptase is usually less than ten times higher than that of beta-tryptase, and the ratio of total to mature tryptase is around 1 if the beta-tryptase level is very high [2].

6.2.1.2 Histamine

Histamine is a biogenic amine synthesised and stored by mast cells and basophils. It is the principal chemical mediator capable of immediate release and resulting in increased vasomotor tone and smooth muscle activity. Mast cells and basophils have a similar capacity to produce histamine [17].

Within cells, histidine decarboxylase acts on histidine to produce histamine. Whilst there are low levels of continuous secretion of histamine, the bulk of the mediator is stored intracellularly. Histamine is bound to proteins and proteoglycans under low pH within granules for secretion. Binding is via carboxyl moieties, plus, possibly, sulphate groups [2].

Rise in anaphylaxis. Just as with tryptase, an increase in urinary or blood tryptase is consistent with anaphylaxis although a normal level does not exclude anaphylaxis having occurred [2].

There is a strong association between elevation in histamine and increasing severity of anaphylactic response. Whilst histamine levels in samples taken with an appropriate methodology have more diagnostic value than tryptase samples, the fact that histamine persists for such a short time in the circulation limits the utility of such quantification in routine clinical practice [27].

6.2.1.3 Metabolites of Histamine

Histamine is mostly metabolically transformed into *N*-methylhistamine within minutes of release, thereafter undergoing conversion to *N*-methylimidazole acetic acid by the action of histamine *N*-methyl transferase and monoamine oxidase, or to imidazole acetic acid by the action of diamine oxidase. *N*-methylhistamine and *N*-methylimidazole acetic acid are formed from breakdown of histamine, whilst imidazole acetic acid is not a histamine breakdown product. Urinary or blood levels of *N*-methylhistamine or *N*-methylimidazole acetic acid are thus associated with the amount of histamine released into the circulation. These metabolites can be potentially found in urine for several hours following an anaphylactic attack. Raised levels of *N*-methylhistamine in urine were noted in specimens taken 6 h after challenge with insect venom in patients who went on to develop systemic anaphylaxis [28].

6.2.2 Prostaglandin and Its Metabolites

Mast cells which have undergone activation, but not basophils, express principally PGD2 as a cyclooxygenase. Antigen-presenting cells, thrombocytes, and Th2 helper cells also secrete the enzyme. PGD2 plays a considerable role in the activation of mast cells and corresponding haemodynamic alterations [29]. As with histamine, systemic clearance occurs rapidly, which renders ascertainment of the elevation in serum PGD2 generally challenging [5]. The principal metabolite of PGD2 is 11β-PGF2α, which is found in the urine. It may have greater sensitivity as a marker of activation for mast cells than *N*-methylhistamine [30–32].

It is of no value to measure PGD2 if the individual is taking drugs that inhibit cyclooxygenase (such as aspirin and similar NSAIDs) since PGD2 synthesis will be inhibited [2].

6.2.3 Chymase and Carboxypeptidase A3

The subset of mast cells known as MCTC produces two proteases: chymase and carboxypeptidase A3. MCTC cells are the dominant mast cell subpopulation intradermally, perivascularly, submucosally, in the heart and in the conjunctiva [33]. The two proteases are stored in secretory granules for export as a macromolecular protease: proteoglycan complex [22]. In post-mortem samples from victims of anaphylaxis, the level of chymase as detected by ELISA was elevated in connection with elevated tryptase levels. By comparison, deaths from other causes were not associated with raised protease levels in serum [34].

6.2.4   5-Levels of Hydroxyindoleacetic Acid

The level of 5-hydroxyindoleacetic acid should be measured in a 24-h urine collection specimen if carcinoid syndrome is suspected [1].

6.3   Confirming the Diagnosis of Anaphylaxis

The main task to be undertaken in the workup of a case of suspected anaphylaxis is confirmation of the clinical suspicion. Anaphylaxis presents with an abrupt onset of symptoms and signs, typically in multiple organ systems, with a time course between several minutes and 2 h [35–40]. There are in excess of 40 different ways that the disorder can manifest [41].

The diagnosis of anaphylaxis is confirmed by a reaction of a type and time course conforming to the pattern of anaphylaxis [35–40]. Although simple in theory, in practice, the diagnosis may be a difficult call, particularly if the episode is hidden. Given that anaphylaxis can result in a fatal outcome [42, 43], patients need to be prepared to treat themselves if there is a risk of recurrence, even where the diagnosis is less than certain. In the case of recurrence, a reassessment is warranted to learn whether the anaphylaxis has had the same trigger on both occasions [42, 43].

6.3.1   History of Exposures and Activities

Clinical history plays a crucial role in diagnosing anaphylaxis, ascertaining the trigger and assessing risk factors that may heighten the probability of severe or potentially fatal anaphylaxis [35].

Every preceding event that resembles anaphylaxis needs to be exhaustively looked at, starting with the 24 h period before symptoms developed, especially focusing on the 1–2 h immediately preceding onset. Key facts may be gleaned from family members, parents, friends, or others who witnessed the event, ambulance crews, and accident and emergency department notekeeping [35].

6.3.2   Exposures

The history needs to list any food or drugs eaten, injections, or in contact with the body. For anaphylaxis in children, adolescents and young adults, an IgE-mediated allergic reaction to food is the most probable cause of anaphylaxis, whilst middle-aged and older adults' episodes are more likely to have been caused by insect venom or medications [35].

6.3.3   Chronology

For it to be likely that a particular trigger caused anaphylaxis, the history will reflect a time sequence compatible with anaphylaxis, particularly with regard to the time between exposure and initial symptoms. Anaphylaxis occurring through IgE develops within minutes to an hour. There are a few exceptions to this general principle, such as anaphylaxis occurring through IgE specific to alpha-1,3-galactose (alpha-gal). In this case, onset may be delayed by 4–6 h after eating the alpha-gal-containing meat [44].

6.3.4   Baseline State of Health and Activities

Information about patients' general health and any exercise undertaken in the 24 h preceding anaphylaxis should be gathered [42, 43, 45]. Of particular relevance are any illnesses and any medication used, such as antipyretics or for menstrual symptoms.

These factors may contribute to patients' susceptibility to anaphylaxis and may modulate the severity of symptoms experienced.

The level of physical exertion should be noted [32, 39, 40, 46]. Exercise can be both the actual trigger for anaphylaxis (exercise-induced asthma, EIA) or worsen the situation when food or drugs are the real cause. In this respect, NSAIDs may be involved. Sometimes, it is a specific foodstuff (e.g. shellfish, wheat, or celery) which, in conjunction with exercise, sets off the anaphylaxis (food-dependent EIA). In some cases, any food item consumed just before activity may set off the anaphylaxis [35].

On rare occasions, sexual activity (kissing or intercourse) may lead to allergenic exposure [40].

6.3.5   Environmental Conditions

Since anaphylaxis may also be triggered by extremes of heat or cold, any unusual environmental conditions should be asked about and noted [40, 46].

6.3.6   Comorbidities

Particular chronic health problems make severe or fatal anaphylaxis more probable [35, 41].

- Asthma, more so if control is suboptimal, raises the risk of severe or fatal anaphylaxis [43, 47, 48].
- Other respiratory or circulatory disorders, such as COPD (chronic obstructive pulmonary disease) or coronary vessel disease, also raise the risk [32, 37, 39, 49, 50].
- Mastocytosis and other lesions of mast cells also have an association with severe or fatal anaphylaxis. Indeed, their existence needs to be diagnostically considered in patients whose anaphylaxis is severe.

References

1. Mustafa SS. Anaphylaxis. In: Kaliner MA, editor. Medscape. http://emedicine.medscape.com/article/135065-overview#showall. Accessed 11 July 2016.
2. Schwartz LB. Laboratory tests to support the clinical diagnosis of anaphylaxis. In: Simons FER, Feldweg AM, editors. Up to Date. http://cursoenarm.net/UPTODATE/contents/mobipreview.htm?13/16/13569?source=see_link. Accessed 11 July 2016.
3. Vadas P, Gold M, Perelman B, et al. Platelet-activating factor, PAF acetylhydrolase, and severe anaphylaxis. N Engl J Med. 2008;358(1):28–35.
4. Schwartz LB, Yunginger JW, Miller J, et al. Time course of appearance and disappearance of human mast cell tryptase in the circulation after anaphylaxis. J Clin Invest. 1989;83:1551.
5. van der Linden PW, Hack CE, Poortman J, et al. Insect-sting challenge in 138 patients: relation between clinical severity of anaphylaxis and mast cell activation. J Allergy Clin Immunol. 1992;90:110.
6. van der Linden PW, Struyvenberg A, Kraaijenhagen RJ, et al. Anaphylactic shock after insect-sting challenge in 138 persons with a previous insect-sting reaction. Ann Intern Med. 1993;118:161.
7. Smith PL, Kagey-Sobotka A, Bleecker ER, et al. Physiologic manifestations of human anaphylaxis. J Clin Invest. 1980;66:1072.
8. Halmerbauer G, Hauk P, Forster J, et al. In vivo histamine release during the first minutes after deliberate sting challenges correlates with the severity of allergic symptoms. Pediatr Allergy Immunol. 1999;10:53.
9. Simons FE. Anaphylaxis. J Allergy Clin Immunol. 2008;121(2 Suppl):S402–7; quiz S420.
10. Akin C. Anaphylaxis and mast cell disease: what is the risk? Curr Allergy Asthma Rep. 2010;10(1):34–8.
11. Bonadonna P, Perbellini O, Passalacqua G, et al. Clonal mast cell disorders in patients with systemic reactions to Hymenoptera stings and increased serum tryptase levels. J Allergy Clin Immunol. 2009;123(3):680–6.
12. Rueff F, Przybilla B, Bilo MB, et al. Predictors of severe systemic anaphylactic reactions in patients with Hymenoptera venom allergy: importance of baseline serum tryptase-a study of the European Academy of Allergology and Clinical Immunology Interest Group on Insect Venom Hypersensitivity. J Allergy Clin Immunol. 2009;124(5):1047–54.
13. Lin RY, Schwartz LB, Curry A, Pesola GR, Knight RJ, Lee HS, et al. Histamine and tryptase levels in patients with acute allergic

reactions: an emergency department-based study. J Allergy Clin Immunol. 2000;106(1 Pt 1):65–71.

14. Simons FE. Anaphylaxis pathogenesis and treatment. Allergy. 2011;66(Suppl 95):31–4.

15. Castells MC, Irani AM, Schwartz LB. Evaluation of human peripheral blood leukocytes for mast cell tryptase. J Immunol. 1987;138:2184.

16. Jogie-Brahim S, Min HK, Fukuoka Y, et al. Expression of alpha-tryptase and beta-tryptase by human basophils. J Allergy Clin Immunol. 2004;113:1086.

17. Schwartz LB, Irani AM, Roller K, et al. Quantitation of histamine, tryptase, and chymase in dispersed human T and TC mast cells. J Immunol. 1987;138:2611.

18. Schwartz LB. Diagnostic value of tryptase in anaphylaxis and mastocytosis. Immunol Allergy Clin N Am. 2006;26:451.

19. Schwartz LB, Min HK, Ren S, et al. Tryptase precursors are preferentially and spontaneously released, whereas mature tryptase is retained by HMC-1 cells, Mono-Mac-6 cells, and human skin-derived mast cells. J Immunol. 2003;170:5667.

20. Caughey GH. Mast cell tryptases and chymases in inflammation and host defense. Immunol Rev. 2007;217:141.

21. Schwartz LB, Bradford TR. Regulation of tryptase from human lung mast cells by heparin. Stabilization of the active tetramer. J Biol Chem. 1986;261:7372.

22. Goldstein SM, Leong J, Schwartz LB, Cooke D. Protease composition of exocytosed human skin mast cell protease-proteoglycan complexes. Tryptase resides in a complex distinct from chymase and carboxypeptidase. J Immunol. 1992;148:2475.

23. Le QT, Min HK, Xia HZ, et al. Promiscuous processing of human alphabeta-protryptases by cathepsins L, B, and C. J Immunol. 2011;186:7136.

24. Pereira PJ, Bergner A, Macedo-Ribeiro S, et al. Human beta-tryptase is a ring-like tetramer with active sites facing a central pore. Nature. 1998;392:306.

25. Schwartz LB, Bradford TR, Rouse C, et al. Development of a new, more sensitive immunoassay for human tryptase: use in systemic anaphylaxis. J Clin Immunol. 1994;14:190.

26. Valent P, Akin C, Arock M, et al. Definitions, criteria and global classification of mast cell disorders with special reference to mast cell activation syndromes: a consensus proposal. Int Arch Allergy Immunol. 2012;157(3):215–25.

27. Laroche D, Vergnaud MC, Dubois F, et al. Plasma histamine and tryptase during anaphylactoid reactions. Agents Actions. 1992;36:C201.

28. Stephan V, Zimmermann A, Kühr J, Urbanek R. Determination of N-methylhistamine in urine as an indicator of histamine release in immediate allergic reactions. J Allergy Clin Immunol. 1990; 86:862.

29. Roberts LJ 2nd, Sweetman BJ, Lewis RA, et al. Increased production of prostaglandin D2 in patients with systemic mastocytosis. N Engl J Med. 1980;303:1400.

30. Awad JA, Morrow JD, Roberts LJ 2nd. Detection of the major urinary metabolite of prostaglandin D2 in the circulation: demonstration of elevated levels in patients with disorders of systemic mast cell activation. J Allergy Clin Immunol. 1994;93:817.

31. Morrow JD, Guzzo C, Lazarus G, et al. Improved diagnosis of mastocytosis by measurement of the major urinary metabolite of prostaglandin D2. J Invest Dermatol. 1995;104:937.

32. Butterfield JH, Weiler CR. Prevention of mast cell activation disorder-associated clinical sequelae of excessive prostaglandin D(2) production. Int Arch Allergy Immunol. 2008;147:338.

33. Schwartz LB. Analysis of MC(T) and MC(TC) mast cells in tissue. Methods Mol Biol. 2006;315:53.

34. Nishio H, Takai S, Miyazaki M, et al. Usefulness of serum mast cell-specific chymase levels for postmortem diagnosis of anaphylaxis. Int J Legal Med. 2005;119:331.

35. Kelso JM. Anaphylaxis: confirming the diagnosis and determining the cause(s). In: Bochner BS, Feldweg AM, editors. Up to Date. http://021081ha8.y.http.www.uptodate.com.proxy.kirikkale-elibrary.com/contents/anaphylaxis-confirming-the-diagnosis-and-determining-the-causes?source=see_link. Accessed 11 July 2016.

36. Simons FE. Anaphylaxis. J Allergy Clin Immunol. 2010;125:S161.

37. Sampson HA, Muñoz-Furlong A, Campbell RL, et al. Second symposium on the definition and management of anaphylaxis: summary report—Second National Institute of Allergy and Infectious Disease/Food Allergy and Anaphylaxis Network symposium. J Allergy Clin Immunol. 2006;117:391.

38. Sampson HA, Muñoz-Furlong A, Bock SA, et al. Symposium on the definition and management of anaphylaxis: summary report. J Allergy Clin Immunol. 2005;115:584.

39. Simons FE, Ardusso LR, Bilò MB, et al. World Allergy Organization anaphylaxis guidelines: summary. J Allergy Clin Immunol. 2011;127:587.

40. Lieberman P, Nicklas RA, Oppenheimer J, et al. The diagnosis and management of anaphylaxis practice parameter: 2010 update. J Allergy Clin Immunol. 2010;126:477.

41. Simons FE. Anaphylaxis, killer allergy: long-term management in the community. J Allergy Clin Immunol. 2006;117:367.

42. Pumphrey RS, Gowland MH. Further fatal allergic reactions to food in the United Kingdom, 1999-2006. J Allergy Clin Immunol. 2007;119:1018.

43. Bock SA, Muñoz-Furlong A, Sampson HA. Further fatalities caused by anaphylactic reactions to food, 2001-2006. J Allergy Clin Immunol. 2007;119:1016.

44. Commins SP, Satinover SM, Hosen J, et al. Delayed anaphylaxis, angioedema, or urticaria after consumption of red meat in patients with IgE antibodies specific for galactose-alpha-1,3-galactose. J Allergy Clin Immunol. 2009;123:426.

45. Summers CW, Pumphrey RS, Woods CN, et al. Factors predicting anaphylaxis to peanuts and tree nuts in patients referred to a specialist center. J Allergy Clin Immunol. 2008;121:632.

46. Robson-Ansley P, Toit GD. Pathophysiology, diagnosis and management of exercise-induced anaphylaxis. Curr Opin Allergy Clin Immunol. 2010;10:312.

47. González-Pérez A, Aponte Z, Vidaurre CF, Rodríguez LA. Anaphylaxis epidemiology in patients with and patients without asthma: a United Kingdom database review. J Allergy Clin Immunol. 2010;125:1098.

48. Iribarren C, Tolstykh IV, Miller MK, Eisner MD. Asthma and the prospective risk of anaphylactic shock and other allergy diagnoses in a large integrated health care delivery system. Ann Allergy Asthma Immunol. 2010;104:371.

49. Triggiani M, Patella V, Staiano RI, et al. Allergy and the cardiovascular system. Clin Exp Immunol. 2008;153(Suppl 1):7.

50. Mueller UR. Cardiovascular disease and anaphylaxis. Curr Opin Allergy Clin Immunol. 2007;7:337.

Chapter 7
Differential Diagnosis for Anaphylaxis

7.1 Introduction

There are a number of frequently encountered conditions that can mimic anaphylaxis. They include acute generalised urticaria, severe angioedema, abrupt deterioration in asthma, fainting, and anxiety or panic attacks. In addition, anaphylaxis can present occasionally as sudden collapse and show no skin signs; hence, it may be mistaken for other conditions presenting as syncope or as threatening syncope. Other potential differential diagnoses include choking and pruritus from external causes, important to consider in the case of neonates and younger children [1–3].

If there is a history of recent exposure to a known allergen, it is straightforward to consider anaphylaxis, even more so if hives and intense itching are present. But if gut symptoms and circulatory compromise are the only presenting symptoms, anaphylaxis springs to mind less readily. In Accident and Emergency Departments, the most common differential diagnoses under consideration are urticaria, anxiety disorders, asthma, fits, and blackouts [4, 5].

© Springer Nature Switzerland AG 2020
C. Cingi, N. B. Muluk, *Quick Guide to Anaphylaxis*,
https://doi.org/10.1007/978-3-030-33639-4_7

7.2   Acute Generalised Urticaria and/or Angioedema

Urticaria and angioedema that begins suddenly and becomes generalised may herald incipient anaphylaxis or may exist as an isolated presentation on its own. In any case, if the urticarial response has been initiated by an allergic reaction to a foodstuff, drug, or insect venom, patients should still use an epinephrine auto-injector to prevent the episode leading to respiratory distress or circulatory compromise [1].

Hives, either with or without accompanying angioedema, affects only the skin and immediately underlying tissues. It may be in connection with other disorders or having a physical trigger such as extreme cold or heat. The factors associated with angioedema, whether allergic or non-allergic, are addressed elsewhere.

Cases of "bradykinin-mediated hereditary or acquired angioedema (C1 inhibitor deficiency)" or "angiotensin-converting enzyme (ACE) inhibitor-induced angioedema" have non-confluent areas of oedema without any accompanying pruritus or erythema. Angioedema affects the deeper layers of the skin or mucosa of the face, the limb extremities, the genitals, and the tongue and larynx, with the potential to cause a life-threatening asphyxic episode. Angioedema can also affect the internal organs, producing a continuous abdominal discomfort ranging in severity from slight discomfort through to vomiting, loose stools, and hypovolaemic circulatory collapse. C4 complement protein is particularly low during attacks of angioedema in the C1 deficiency disorder, but is also low between attacks, too. The inhibition of C1-esterase either does not occur, or only occurs at very low levels in many sufferers from this condition [6–8]. Anaphylaxis usually progresses to involve multiple organ systems apart from just the skin and mucosal surfaces, so if pruritus and urticaria begin to occur, it is essential for the treating physician to identify these signs and link them to a probable allergen trigger, if one is found to have been encountered in the minutes or hours preceding an anaphylactic attack [1–3, 9].

7.3 Asthma Exacerbation

Both an acute asthma attack and anaphylaxis may present acutely as wheezing, coughing, and dyspnoea. Thus, if any patient does show these signs, and in addition, urticaria, erythema, angioedema, hoarseness, laryngeal constriction and abdominal pain, vomiting, loose stools, vertigo, syncope, or hypotension, the diagnosis of anaphylaxis needs to be contemplated. Similarly, if patients develop symptoms within the appropriate time frame to known or suspected allergic triggers, such as certain foods, drugs, or insect venoms, anaphylaxis needs to be excluded [1, 2, 10].

7.4 Vasovagal Syncope

Vasovagal episodes are the most commonly encountered anaphylaxis mimics. A vasovagal episode consists of a reflex arc becoming overactive within the parasympathetic nervous system, resulting in profound cardiac slowing, dilation of blood vessels and hypotension. Other terms applied to this phenomenon of fainting include situational syncope, vasovagal syncope, and vasodepression. It is characterised by low BP, pallor, weakness, nausea, reflux, and hyperhidrosis. The usual triggers are physical or emotional stress. Bradycardia is a cardinal feature. Since similar symptoms may appear in an anaphylactic response, the fact that there is no bronchospastic response, there is a lack of erythema and a difference in the appearance of the skin should help to inform the differential diagnosis [5].

Fainting may occur as part of an anaphylactic response or may occur on its own. The usual vasovagal loss of consciousness has the features outlined above and may be treated by laying the patient down flat [1].

One notable difference from an anaphylactic episode is that in anaphylaxis there will usually be abrupt onset of erythema rather than pallor, plus symptoms that are not part of a vasovagal response will coexist, such as acute paraesthesia, urticarial rash, angioedema, hoarseness and laryngeal constriction, stridor, wheezing, coughing, dyspnoea, abdominal pain, or diarrhoea. Tachycardia is a much more usual response than bradycardia in anaphylactic responses [1, 2, 10].

7.5 Panic Attack/Acute Anxiety

In panic attacks (sudden onset of severe anxiety), the symptoms include a sense of impending doom, dyspnoea, flushing, diaphoresis, tremor, cardiac palpitations, globus hystericus (an imagined blockage in the throat), abdominal symptoms, lightheadedness, abdominodynia, and numb sensations in the limbs [2, 10].

Whilst there is a degree of overlap with the symptomatology of anaphylaxis, the typical panic attack does not have the features of urticaria, angioedema, hoarseness, stridor, wheezing and coughing, profoundly low BP or syncope, unlike anaphylaxis [1–3].

7.6 Other Causes of Sudden Collapse

Anaphylaxis may on occasion present as an abrupt loss of consciousness, with absent cutaneous findings, which may lead to diagnostic uncertainty. A differential diagnosis for sudden collapse is broad and should consider potentially fatal conditions such as acute myocardial infarction, dysrhythmia, complications of aortic stenosis or hypertrophic cardiomyopathies, pulmonary embolism, profound haemorrhage (e.g. gastrointestinal haemorrhage or rupture caused by an ectopic pregnancy), dissection of the aorta, subarachnoid haemorrhage, and certain other conditions. An elevation in tryptase is found in both anaphylaxis and from necrotic cardiac muscle tissue [2, 3, 11–15]. Thus, if a patient suddenly collapses, a clear history and relevant investigations, such as ECG, are of the utmost importance in reaching a correct assessment of aetiology [1].

7.7   Other Causes of Acute Respiratory Distress

Some potential causes of acute respiratory distress include vocal cord dysfunction, choking or aspiration of a foreign body, aspiration pneumonia, pneumothorax, or inflammation of the epiglottis [1].

7.7.1   Vocal Cord Dysfunction

Vocal cord dysfunction entails the vocal cords closing when breath is indrawn, contrary to the usual physiology. Shortness of breath, coughing, stridor when breathing in or wheezing when breathing out may be seen. It is mostly seen in young girls although there are reports of its occurrence in adults as well as children generally [16, 17]. The diagnosis can be made by directly visualising the abnormal action of the vocal cords using a laryngoscope [1].

7.8   Flushing Syndromes

Various medications or agents are known to produce flushing, such as histamine, callicrein, neuropeptides, nicotine, and ACE inhibitors. It is also found in carcinoid syndrome [18], where the usual presentation is erythema, loose stools, griping abdominal pain, and wheeze. A further key differential to consider is a medullary thyroid carcinoma (producing erythema facially, on the extremities and telangiectasia. It is often an inherited condition). Flushing disorders can be divided into "wet" and "dry" subtypes. Wet subtype flushing features diaphoresis as a result of sympathetic system activation of sweat glands, as can happen in the menopause or after eating pungent foods. In the dry subtype, diaphoresis is absent. This is the type seen in carcinoid syndrome. Alcohol may produce a similar syndrome, notably amongst people of Asian extraction who have a congenital lack of aldehyde dehydrogenase. Alcohol may also trigger erythema in cases of Hodgkin's lymphoma, hypereosinophilia, and in splenectomised individuals. Each of these needs to be considered in taking a history of a possible anaphylactic episode. An autonomic epileptic attack may also involve profound alterations in blood pressure, flushing, fainting, and tachycardia [5].

7.9   Tumours

Various neoplasms may produce flushing, including carcinoids, gut malignancies, medullary thyroid, renal cell, and pancreatic. A few such neoplasms are discussed below [1]:

7.9.1   Carcinoid Tumours

Carcinoid syndrome is a term describing the syndromic occurrence of a number of symptoms related to the discharge of 5-hydroxytryptamine (5-HT), substance P and other vasoactive mediators by carcinoid neoplasms of the small intestine, appendix, and large intestine. Profuse erythema occurs in many cases, typically facially, over the neck and upper torso. The affected areas range in colour from red to purple, and there may be mild sensory disturbance in the affected zones. Flushing begins abruptly and has a duration of 20–30 s although over time flushing periods may lengthen in duration. Loose stools are characteristic, and wheezing is sometimes observed [19, 20]. If carcinoid is suspected, blood levels of 5-HT and a 24 h collection for the urinary metabolite 5-HIAA (5-hydroxyindoleacetic acid) should be performed, alongside dietary exclusion of 5-HT and tryptophan-rich foodstuffs [1].

7.9.2 Gastrointestinal Tumours

Neoplasms within the gut that secrete vasointestinal polypeptide (VIP) or substance P are extremely uncommon. The majority of such cases produce very loose stools and have hypokalaemia with hypochlorhydria, and a small number (1 in 5) experience flushing episodes. Blood levels for VIP or substance P are beneficial diagnostically [1, 19].

7.9.3 Medullary Carcinoma of the Thyroid

This malignancy is usually found as a solitary thyroid nodule seen in a middle-aged patient. Erythema affecting the face and diarrhoea may happen in late stage disease [1, 19].

7.10 Postprandial Syndromes

Simple scombroid (due to a histamine-like toxin) occurs in adults and children. If fish are incorrectly stored and preserved, enterobacteria may colonise the fish, producing large volumes of histamine by bacterial metabolism of histidine. Usually *Klebsiella oxytoca* and *Morganella morganii* are the organisms responsible. If children present with severe hives and headache, vomiting, and nausea after a meal, scombroid poisoning should be considered [21]. Patients on Isoniazid are particularly susceptible [22]. Diagnosis is more straightforward if cases present together in Accident and Emergency having consumed the same infected fish. A peculiar feature of the disorder is the serological rise in histamine without an accompanying rise in tryptase [5].

Monosodium glutamate (a common ingredient in Chinese takeaways) can also give rise to erythema, headache, and GI disturbance. Signs and symptoms include chest pain, facial oedema, erythema, pins and needles, diaphoresis, headaches, palpitations, and nausea with or without actual vomiting [22]. An identical picture may happen from ingesting sulphites, which may be added to gelatine, sauces, wine, fruit juices, or shellfish. The syndrome starts between 1 and 14 h after eating the affected food [5].

7.10.1　Scombroidosis

Scombroid syndrome (aka histamine food poisoning) is seen 15 min to 1 h after eating spoilt fish, such as mackerel, sardines, anchovies, or herrings. Flushes begin abruptly, with accompanying headache, nausea, vomiting, diarrhoea, abdominal discomfort, difficulty swallowing, palpitations, vertigo, and profoundly low BP. Hives and pruritus also occur [1, 23].

The syndrome is a result of histamine produced in fish that have been improperly stored and refrigerated, where bacteria found in muscle tissue of the spoilt fish decarboxylate L-histidine, producing histamine. Cooking has no effect on histamine levels. A clue to the diagnosis occurs when there are a group of related cases with a history of eating fish from the same source [1, 2, 10].

It is possible to differentiate scombroidosis from allergy by skin prick testing and serological quantification of specific IgE to fish. If allergic in aetiology, prick tests will be positive and IgE will be raised, but if scombroidosis is the reason, these tests will be negative [1, 24].

7.10.2　Anisakiasis

Anisakis simplex is a parasite found in fish. Its presence in fish may cause an anaphylactic response through an allergic response. A typical history is of eating raw or half-raw sea fish 1 or 2 h before the attack. Marinated anchovies may be the problem. Skin prick tests are positive for the parasite, and specific IgE is raised. The main allergic epitope is Ani s 7. Commercially prepared skin prick test concentrates and specific IgE to the fish as a whole are usually negative [1, 25, 26].

7.10.3   Pollen-Food Allergy Syndrome

Pollen-food allergy syndrome is also known as oral allergy syndrome. It typically occurs in individuals suffering from allergic rhinoconjunctivitis or dust allergy. The disorder occurs when there is cross-reactivity for dust antigens with uncooked leafy vegetables or plant proteins in nuts. The antigens are often profilins or lipid transfer proteins. The usual cross-reactivity with dust antigens occurs with apple, carrot, kiwi, celery, or pear, whilst melon or banana stimulates ragweed allergic patients. Potatoes, tomatoes, watermelon, or kiwi may cross-react with grass pollen. The symptoms seen are paraesthesiae, lingual and labial angioedema, altered taste sensation, throat tightness, and ear pain. It only occurs if the food is raw [27, 28]. Some dust allergy sufferers may have an anaphylactic response [1].

7.10.4   Food Poisoning

Food poisoning is brought about either by microbial contamination of food or by the toxins produced by microbes in the food. The presentation may be one of vomiting accompanied by griping stomach pains occurring within 2 h of eating the poisoned food. Generally speaking, food poisoning does not produce symptoms beyond the gut itself [1].

7.10.5   Caustic Ingestion (Young Children)

Young children may sometimes accidentally swallow corrosive substances, and this may mimic the appearances of anaphylaxis since it may lead to nausea, vomiting, dysphagia and labial, lingual, and pharyngeal oedema [29]. The swallowing may be unwitnessed or care givers may fail to give a history out of a fear of possible negative consequences for themselves. Clues to the diagnosis come from the lack of previous hypersensitivity reactions of any kind (including to food), and non-response to treatment given for supposed anaphylaxis. Imaging with the endoscope or laryngoscope will usually reveal ulcerated mucosa within the upper airway and oesophagus [1].

7.11   Other Causes of Shock

In hypovolaemic shock, loose stools and griping abdominal pain may always occur, but there will usually be no skin symptoms. On balance, it is not particularly challenging to distinguish between septic and cardiogenic aetiologies since septic shock is usually accompanied by fever, whereas cardiogenic shock is associated with pre-existing cardiac conditions [5, 30].

7.12   Excess Histamine Syndromes

Overproduction of histamine may occur due to mast cell proliferative disorders, some leukaemic subtypes and surgical rupture of an hydatid cyst [1].

Rare conditions may sometimes influence the severity of an anaphylactic episode. Severe promyelocytic leukaemia and basophilic leukaemia are rare conditions, in which systemic tretinoin treatment may precipitate an anaphylactic reaction [31]. Histamine release in response to echinococcus infestation is another possible trigger to anaphylaxis [32]. The so-called red man syndrome is linked to vancomycin usage. Intravenous administration of this antibiotic can activate mast cells even without a prior sensitisation event [5, 33].

7.13   Nonorganic Diseases

There are certain psychological disorders that may have the appearances of anaphylaxis. In factitious disorder (Munchausen Syndrome), stridor may be heard, which may mimic that seen in anaphylaxis [34]. Globus hystericus and panic attacks may also act as anaphylaxis mimics. Vocal cord dysfunction is frequent in young paediatric cases and may look like an anaphylactic episode [5, 35].

7.13.1   Munchausen Stridor

Some cases of factitious disorder (in which patients knowingly feign physical symptoms to garner sympathy) present very similarly to cases of vocal cord dysfunction. They may be willing to adduct their vocal cords when desired to do so and asking them to cough may uncover the subterfuge [1].

Munchausen-associated anaphylaxis is genuine anaphylaxis, but intentionally produced by the patient through willingly eating food or drugs to which they know they are allergic [1, 36, 37].

7.14   Rare Disorders

7.14.1   Pheochromocytoma

Pheochromocytoma is a catecholaminergic neoplasm arising from cells of the adrenal medulla and produces a syndrome of long-standing headache, diaphoresis, and elevated heart rate. Hypertension is far more usual than paradoxical hypotension.

Patients tend to be pale in appearance rather than flushed. Initial workup in a case where the history suggests pheochromocytoma includes 24-h urine collection for quantification of the adrenal metabolites metadrenaline, and other catecholamines [1].

7.14.2   Capillary Leak Syndrome

"Idiopathic systemic capillary leak syndrome" is a rare disorder with a high associated mortality, in which angioedema recurs frequently alongside gut symptoms, and shock alongside haemoconcentration. It is usually found in association with a monoclonal gammopathy. An elevated haematocrit alongside hypotension may raise clinical suspicions. It is treated aggressively by fluid resuscitation and supportive measures [1, 38, 39].

7.15   Miscellaneous

Hereditary angioedema, which produces oedema in the skin and submucosae and respiratory and gut symptoms. May look similar to anaphylaxis [40]. When they appear in Accident and Emergency, there is usually an attack triggered by dental examinations or mouth checkups. The overall prevalence is 1 in 50,000. It is important to recognise such attacks for what they are at the onset as 15–30% of sufferers will have a fatal episode. Mostly, however, diagnosis of hereditary angioedema is relatively straightforward [5].

Systemic capillary leak syndrome is a grave condition that may prove fatal and features severe angioedema, excessive thirst, oliguria, or anuria [41]. Extremely high levels of IL-2 have occasionally been reported to occur. Gleich's syndrome causes a florid hypereosinophilia (reaching blood levels of 60,000–70,000/μL), with enormous expansion in serological titres of immunoglobulins A and E. The severity of symptoms is dictated by the level of eosinophilia since eosinophilic degranulation is the root cause of its clinical manifestations [5, 42].

References

1. Kelso JM. Differential diagnosis of anaphylaxis in children and adults. In: Bochner BS, Felsdweg AM, editors. UpToDate. http://www.uptodate.com/contents/differential-diagnosis-of-anaphylaxis-in-children-and-adults. Accessed 12 July 2016.

2. Simons FE, Ardusso LR, Bilò MB, et al. World allergy organization guidelines for the assessment and management of anaphylaxis. World Allergy Organ J. 2011;4:13.

3. Simons FE, Frew AJ, Ansotegui IJ, et al. Risk assessment in anaphylaxis: current and future approaches. J Allergy Clin Immunol. 2007;120:S2.

4. Simons FE, Frew AJ, Ansotegui IJ, et al. Practical allergy (PRACTALL) report: risk assessment in anaphylaxis. Allergy. 2008;63:35–7.

5. Martelli A, Ghiglioni D, Sarratud T, Calcinai E, Veehof S, Terracciano L, Fiocchi A. Anaphylaxis in the emergency department: a paediatric perspective: differential diagnosis. Medscape. http://www.medscape.org/viewarticle/583328_4. Accessed 12 July 2016.

6. Zuraw BL. Clinical practice. Hereditary angioedema. N Engl J Med. 2008;359:1027.

7. Levy JH, Freiberger DJ, Roback J. Hereditary angioedema: current and emerging treatment options. Anesth Analg. 2010;110:1271.

8. Bork K, Hardt J, Witzke G. Fatal laryngeal attacks and mortality in hereditary angioedema due to C1-INH deficiency. J Allergy Clin Immunol. 2012;130:692.

9. Sampson HA, Muñoz-Furlong A, Campbell RL, et al. Second symposium on the definition and management of anaphylaxis: summary report—Second National Institute of Allergy and Infectious Disease/Food Allergy and Anaphylaxis Network symposium. J Allergy Clin Immunol. 2006;117:391.

10. Lieberman PL. Anaphylaxis. In: Adkinson Jr NF, Bochner BS, Busse WW, et al., editors. Middleton's allergy: principles and practice. 7th ed. St. Louis: Mosby; 2009. p. 1027.

11. Worm M, Edenharter G, Ruëff F, et al. Symptom profile and risk factors of anaphylaxis in Central Europe. Allergy. 2012;67:691.

12. Palmiere C, Comment L, Vilarino R, et al. Measurement of β-tryptase in postmortem serum in cardiac deaths. J Forensic Legal Med. 2014;23:12.

13. Triggiani M, Patella V, Staiano RI, et al. Allergy and the cardiovascular system. Clin Exp Immunol. 2008;153(Suppl 1):7.

14. Triggiani M, Montagni M, Parente R, Ridolo E. Anaphylaxis and cardiovascular diseases: a dangerous liaison. Curr Opin Allergy Clin Immunol. 2014;14:309.

15. Campbell RL, Hagan JB, Li JT, et al. Anaphylaxis in emergency department patients 50 or 65 years or older. Ann Allergy Asthma Immunol. 2011;106:401.
16. Noyes BE, Kemp JS. Vocal cord dysfunction in children. Paediatr Respir Rev. 2007;8:155.
17. Bahrainwala AH, Simon MR. Wheezing and vocal cord dysfunction mimicking asthma. Curr Opin Pulm Med. 2001;7:8.
18. Aldrich LB, Moattari R, Vinik AL. Distinguishing features of idiopathic flushing and carcinoid syndromes. Arch Intern Med. 1988;148:2614–8.
19. Izikson L, English JC 3rd, Zirwas MJ. The flushing patient: differential diagnosis, workup, and treatment. J Am Acad Dermatol. 2006;55:193.
20. Kulke MH, Mayer RJ. Carcinoid tumors. N Engl J Med. 1999;340:858.
21. Lieberman P. Anaphylaxis. Med Clin N Am. 2006;90:77–95.
22. Settipane GA. The restaurant syndromes. Arch Intern Med. 1986;146:2614–8.
23. Becker K, Southwick K, Reardon J, et al. Histamine poisoning associated with eating tuna burgers. JAMA. 2001;285:1327.
24. Ricci G, Zannoni M, Cigolini D, et al. Tryptase serum level as a possible indicator of scombroid syndrome. Clin Toxicol (Phila). 2010;48:203.
25. AAITO-IFIACI Anisakis Consortium. Anisakis hypersensitivity in Italy: prevalence and clinical features: a multicenter study. Allergy. 2011;66:1563.
26. Rodríguez E, Anadón AM, García-Bodas E, et al. Novel sequences and epitopes of diagnostic value derived from the Anisakis simplex Ani s 7 major allergen. Allergy. 2008;63:219.
27. Webber CM, England RW. Oral allergy syndrome: a clinical, diagnostic, and therapeutic challenge. Ann Allergy Asthma Immunol. 2010;104:101.
28. Pascal M, Muñoz-Cano R, Reina Z, et al. Lipid transfer protein syndrome: clinical pattern, cofactor effect and profile of molecular sensitization to plant-foods and pollens. Clin Exp Allergy. 2012;42:1529.
29. Sherenian MG, Clee M, Schondelmeyer AC, et al. Caustic ingestions mimicking anaphylaxis: case studies and literature review. Pediatrics. 2015;135:e547.
30. Lieberman P. Anaphylaxis and anaphylactoid reactions. In: Middleton Jr E, editor. Allergy: principles and practice. 5th ed. St. Louis: Mosby; 1998. p. 1079–92.
31. Koike T, Tatewaki W, Aoki A. Brief report: severe symptoms of hyperhistaminemia after the treatment of acute promyelocytic leukemia with tretinoin. N Engl J Med. 1992;327:385–7.

32. Wellhoener P, Weitz G, Bechstein W, et al. Severe anaphylactic shock in a patient with a cystic liver lesion. Intensive Care Med. 2000;26:1578.
33. Sivagnanam S, Deleu D. Red man syndrome. Crit Care. 2003;7:119–20.
34. Patterson R, Schatz M. Factitious allergic emergencies: anaphylaxis and laryngeal edema. J Allergy Clin Immunol. 1975;56:152–9.
35. Goodman DL, O'Connel MA, Sklarew PR. Vocal cord dysfunction presenting as anaphylaxis. J Allergy Clin Immunol. 1991;87:278.
36. Greenberger PA, Lieberman P. Idiopathic anaphylaxis. J Allergy Clin Immunol Pract. 2014;2:243.
37. Bahna SL, Oldham JL. Munchausen stridor-a strong false alarm of anaphylaxis. Allergy Asthma Immunol Res. 2014;6:577.
38. Druey KM, Greipp PR. Narrative review: the systemic capillary leak syndrome. Ann Intern Med. 2010;153:90.
39. Dowden AM, Rullo OJ, Aziz N, et al. Idiopathic systemic capillary leak syndrome: novel therapy for acute attacks. J Allergy Clin Immunol. 2009;124:1111.
40. Gompels MM, Lock RJ, Abinun M, et al. C1 inhibitor deficiency: consensus document. Clin Exp Immunol. 2005;139:379–94.
41. Sahnoun I, Harmouche H, Aouni M, et al. Systemic Capillary Leak Syndrome: two case reports. Rev Int Med. 2005;26:409–14.
42. Gleich GJ. Episodic angioedema associated with eosinophilia. N Engl J Med. 1984;310:1621–6.

Chapter 8
Treatment of Anaphylaxis

8.1 Introduction

Anaphylaxis is a clinical emergency that necessitates recognition and treatment without delay. The necessary equipment and medications to treat the condition must be easily at hand in clinical settings. Lieberman et al. have described the set-up required in a very thorough way [1–6].

Patients within the community who are developing signs of a severe anaphylactic response should first be treated following a standardised protocol. High flow oxygen, cardiac monitoring, and the establishment of venous access are amongst the first measures to be taken. Even if symptoms are not present, but there has been a previous anaphylactic tendency in the patient, and now re-exposure has occurred, these measures are appropriate. If only symptoms of a localised allergic response occur, intervention need not progress beyond basic life support (BLS) [1].

How anaphylactic responses need to be treated depends on the severity of the unfolding reaction, and how responsive the patient is to various countermeasures. If no threat to life is observed, a 4–6 h observation may be all that is needed. But for those whose reactions are resistant to intervention or whose anaphylaxis

© Springer Nature Switzerland AG 2020
C. Cingi, N. B. Muluk, *Quick Guide to Anaphylaxis*,
https://doi.org/10.1007/978-3-030-33639-4_8

threatens respiratory and circulatory collapse, remaining under prolonged observation either in Accident and Emergency or an observation unit will be appropriate [1].

8.2   Accident and Emergency Department Interventions

A number of different elements in clinical management need to be carefully co-ordinated [7–13]:

- The initial assessment should focus on ABC (airway, breathing, circulation) and consciousness level. Physical examination should concentrate on the presence or absence of angioedema in the oropharynx, lips, and tongue. The patient should speak (e.g. say his/her name) to allow assessment of epiglottitis. Cutaneous examination for hives and angioedema needs to be performed. If they are found, this gives support to a diagnosis of anaphylaxis [7].
- Adrenaline should be administered i.m. into the mid to outer region of the thigh [14–21]. If a severe reaction is anticipated, i.v. adrenaline should be at hand [7].
- Provided there is no oedema within the upper airway, patients should be reclined to permit sufficient circulation to the essential organs. Pregnant women should be laid on their left side to prevent obstruction of venous return by the uterine contents [22]. Lying down helps to reduce the effects of developing hypotension and impaired cardiac venous return, leading to cardiac failure. Such an occurrence can cause death almost instantly [19]. Patients whose breathing is severely laboured or who are vomiting may be unable to cope with being supine and need to be put in a comfortable position with their feet up if at all possible [7].
- Additional oxygen, initially through a non-rebreather mask at a rate of 15 L/min or commercially available breathing sets which supply between 70 and 100% oxygen, should be provided [7].

- Dual intravenous access via large-diameter catheter (ideally 14–16 gauge in the majority of adults) needs to be established in case rapid fluid resuscitation becomes necessary. If it is not possible to obtain venous access in a timely fashion, intraosseous routes should be considered [7].
- If an adult patient is maintaining his/her blood pressure, the venous access should be kept open by supplying 125 mL isotonic saline (0.9%) over 1 h. For children maintaining their BP, the rate at which isotonic saline is delivered is based on their bulk [7].
- Throughout the anaphylactic attack, there needs to be constant monitoring of the cardiovascular and respiratory systems, including heart load, BP, cardiac rate, respiratory rate, and oxygen saturation via pulse oximetry [7].

8.2.1   Management of the Airway

At the very beginning, the airway should be carefully checked. If it is needed, insert an artificial airway and consider adding mechanical ventilation. Assess the consciousness level and measure BP, pulse rate, and oxygen saturation. Lie the patient down flat and keep the legs up high, whilst providing oxygen. Airway management can prove of utmost importance. One of the easiest and fastest ways to support breathing is by provision of a mask with a one-way valve and a port to supply oxygen (e.g. Pocket-Mask [Laerdal Medical Corporation, Gatesville, TX] or similar devices). Ventilating the patient with supplemental oxygen in this way has been shown to produce saturation levels on a par with endotracheal intubation. If patient breathing is not very laboured, they should be able to breathe freely through the mask [1].

Standard rapid sequence induction (RSI) systems are in use but their use may result in the airway not being maintained in cases with significant airway-associated oedema. The development of severe oedema within the larynx may preclude endotracheal intubation in some cases of anaphylaxis. Adrenaline may rapidly restore the airway, but if it fails to do so, endotracheal intubation will be the only option. Whilst oedema is resolving, it may be acceptable to continue ventilation with a bag and mask [1].

Under exceptional circumstances, where endotracheal intubation and bag and ventilatory mask options are both unavailable, a cricothyrotomy may be the only way to prevent loss of life. Cricothyrotomy is preferable to emergency tracheotomy as the procedure is more straightforward to accomplish [1].

Wheeze or stridor suggest spasticity of the bronchi or oedematous mucosae. Adrenaline and inhaled beta agonist administration is effective in reducing both. Inhaled beta agonists can prevent spasm of the bronchi and should be advised to all cases where there is a complaint of wheeze. It has been suggested that persistent bronchospasm may be treated with steroids, on the analogy of their beneficial role in reversing airway tightening in asthma and COPD. As in asthma treatment, the onset of benefit occurs after a few hours. Aminophylline has also been used to treat anaphylactic attacks and may have a more rapid onset of action than steroids [1].

In bradykinin-mediated angioedema (including angioedema secondary to the use of ACE inhibitor drugs), antihistamines and corticosteroids have a more limited role and adrenaline may be needed for severe episodes, with the likelihood that active management of the airway will also be required [1].

8.2.2   Cardiac Monitoring

It is essential to use a heart monitor when anaphylaxis is severe or pre-existent cardiac disease is present, even more so when treatment involves adrenergic agonists. Pulse oximetry has a key role, too [1].

8.2.3   Intravenous Access

Since a high volume of intravenous fluids may be necessary for resuscitation, large bore cannulae should be used. Isotonic crystalloids (such as isotonic saline or Ringer's lactate) are preferable. If skin signs are the only feature of a reaction, a flow rate sufficient to keep the line open will suffice. If the patient develops tachycardia or low BP, a bolus of fluid can be injected (20 mg/kg for a child, 1 L for adults). Further management then depends upon individual response. Large amounts of fluid may be necessitated where hypotension is severe [1].

8.2.4 Pharmacological Treatments

Anaphylaxis varies considerably in severity and is hard to predict. It ranges from reactions of a mild character that resolve spontaneously to a reaction that proves severe, leading to respiratory and circulatory shutdown and death [23]. It is a practical impossibility to predict at the outset the severity of an anaphylactic reaction, how quickly it may progress and the degree to which it will abate, given that so many factors influencing individual reactions remain unknown. For this reason, timely administration of intramuscular adrenaline is of the utmost importance to prevent the progression to a life-threatening condition [7].

8.2.4.1 Adrenaline

Mechanisms of Action of Adrenaline

Adrenaline has an ability to influence the pathophysiological mechanisms of anaphylaxis that exceeds that of any other agent. It inhibits mast cell degranulation [24], inhibits or ameliorates the narrowing of the airway in its upper and lower portions and reverses circulatory shutdown [7]:

- Action as an α1-adrenergic agonist—vasoconstrictive, leading to an increase in the resistance of the peripheral vasculature and decrease in the oedema gathered in the mucosae, such as the upper section of the airway.
- β1 adrenergic agonist actions—more powerful heart contractions and alteration in cardiac rate

- $\beta 2$ adrenergic agonist actions—dilatation of bronchi and decreased mast cell and basophil discharge [7].

Adverse Effects of Adrenaline

At all ages, adrenaline at small doses creates a mild and short-lived feeling of anxiety, agitation, and can give rise to headaches, feeling unsteady, experiencing palpitations, appearance of pallor and tremor [16, 25–27]. This picture is the same as that occurs during the "fight-or-flight" response, in which there is endogenous release of adrenaline caused by a terrifying or life-threatening situation [7].

Rarely, adrenaline may precipitate a ventricular dysrhythmia, angina pectoris, necrosis of myocardial tissue, pulmonary oedema, abrupt peaks in BP and even intracranial haemorrhage. However, anaphylaxis alone may produce angina pectoris, necrosis of myocardium, and cardiac rhythmic abnormalities, even without the administration of exogenous adrenaline [28].

For the most part, severe side effects are linked to giving adrenaline as an intravenous bolus, particularly if the dosage is too high [7, 14, 25, 29, 30].

Dosing and Administration

Adrenaline is commercially available in a variety of doses. It is essential to use the correct concentration to avoid the potential for cardiac complications that may occur with the drug [8–12]. There is still no full consensus amongst physicians as to the best adrenaline regimen for the treatment of anaphylaxis [29–31].

Intramuscular Epinephrine Injection

In most cases, the best way to administer adrenaline in anaphylaxis is via intramuscular injection. The intramuscular route is preferable to subcutaneous injection since it more rapidly results in a rise in circulating adrenaline and ensures more even organ distribution [17, 18]. Intramuscular injections have a lower risk of inducing ventricular dysrhythmias and severe hypertensive episodes than intravenous bolus injection. Adrenaline for intramuscular use is at a concentration of 1 mg/mL, corresponding to 1:1000 [7].

IM dosage—If it is possible to prepare and administer precisely calculated amounts of adrenaline, the dose should be 0.01 mg/kg patient weight (to a maximum dosage of 0.5 mg) on each occasion and the injection site is the vastus lateralis muscle on the lateral aspect of the thigh. The injection should be drawn up using a 1 mL capacity syringe and a solution of 1 mg/mL adrenaline [7].

If the dosage needs to be guessed at [7]:

- Infants and younger children below 15 kg should receive a precisely calculated amount based on their body mass, rather than an estimate, wherever practicable to do so. Where the calculation of a precise dose would cause a significant delay in administering relief to a child entering a rapidly worsening episode, a risk-benefit assessment of just using a 0.15 mg auto-injector instead needs to be undertaken. Usually the resulting circulating adrenaline level only causes short-lived and moderate symptoms [32].
- Children with a weight between 15 and 29 kg may have 0.15 mg (0.15 mL of a 1 mg/mL solution) administered [33].
- Patients with a weight between 30 and 50 kg may have 0.3 mg (0.3 mL of a 1 mg/mL solution) administered [7].
- Patients with a weight exceeding 50 kg may have 0.5 mg (0.5 mL of a 1 mg/mL solution) administered. For obese patients, a 1.5-inch needle can be used to enter the muscle below the subcutaneous fat layer [7].

Adrenaline Auto-Injectors

An auto-injector can also be used to deliver adrenaline intramuscularly. They come in 0.15 and 0.3 mg dosages. Children who weigh between 10 and 29 kg need the 0.15 mg dose, whereas those over 30 kg will require the 0.3 mg dose auto-injector [7].

Currently, adrenaline by intramuscular injection is the treatment of choice for anaphylaxis [34, 35]. Outside hospitals, adrenaline (epinephrine) auto-injectors (EAI) are the usual way of providing adrenaline. In North America, the Epipen® [36] and

Auvi-Q® [37] (Allerject® in Canada [38]) are currently the most popular EAI for physicians to prescribe [39].

The Epipen Jr® and the Auvi-Q®/Allerject® 0.15 mg are specifically intended to be used in children at risk of anaphylaxis whose weight is from 15 to 30 kg. In Europe, Jext® and Emerade® are available. They each deliver a 0.15 mg dose. For patients whose weight is above 30 kg, Epipen® and Auvi-Q®/Allerject® 0.30 mg are suitable. In Europe, Jext and Emerade® are available with identical doses. Emerade® is also available in a 0.5 mg dose to treat adults [39].

A selection of adrenaline auto-injectors and their specifications are outlined below [39]:

- Epipen Jr®, Auvi-Q®/Allerject®: Dosage: 0.15 mg; needle length: 12.7 mm; distance between skin and muscle: 10.7 mm
- Epipen®Auvi-Q®/Allerject®: Dosage: 0.3 mg; needle length: 15.2 mm; distance between skin and muscle: 13.2 mm
- Jext® 0.15 mg: Dosage: 0.15 mg; needle length: 15.7 mm; distance between skin and muscle: 13.7 mm
- Jext® 0.3 mg: Dosage: 0.3 mg; needle length: 15.7 mm; distance between skin and muscle: 13.7 mm
- Emerade® 0.15 mg: Dosage: 0.15 mg; needle length: 16 mm; distance between skin and muscle: 14 mm
- Emerade® 0.3 mg: Dosage: 0.3 mg; needle length: 23 mm; distance between skin and muscle: 21 mm
- Emerade® 0.5 mg: Dosage: 0.5 mg; needle length: 23 mm; distance between skin and muscle: 21 mm

Intravenous Bolus of Adrenaline (To Be Avoided or Used Only Cautiously)

Intravenous bolus delivery of adrenaline is linked to the majority of the mistakes occurring in dosing adrenaline and with the circulatory complications that do not usually occur if instead a gradual ongoing infusion is set up. It should be avoided wherever possible [14, 25, 29, 30]. A gradual infusion may be chosen in cases where intramuscular injections have been ineffective [10, 40]. An observational study of 301 cases attending Accident and Emergency for anaphylaxis and given adrenaline found four instances of excessive dose usage, in each case involving intravenous bolus administration [30]. Adverse cardiovascular events had a higher likelihood of occurring with i.v. Bolus than with either gradual intravenous infusions or intramuscular routes of delivery. Adverse events in these categories happened in 4 out of 30, 0 out of 4, and 3 out of 245 cases, respectively [7].

8.2.4.2   Administration of Antihistamines and Corticosteroids

Treating anaphylaxis in the standard way involves utilising antihistamines and corticosteroids alongside adrenaline. However, since antihistamines act more slowly than adrenaline and do not help control BP, reliance on them as sole agent is ill-advised [41]. Rather, antihistamines should be used in conjunction with adrenaline [1].

It is preferable to co-administer agents that blockade both H1 and H2 receptors, as the combination has been found to be superior to single type blockade for reduction of histaminergic symptomatology. A suitable combination is diphenhydramine and ranitidine. Giving these agents intravenously helps to counter the otherwise problematic shifts in intestinal and intramuscular absorption that can arise from haemodynamic changes in anaphylaxis. If a reaction is relatively mild, it may be possible still to rely on oral or intramuscular administration [1].

Corticosteroids lack an acute action in anaphylaxis [42]. However, they should be given in a timely fashion so as to prevent a biphasic-pattern anaphylaxis from occurring. Individuals with asthma and certain other conditions who have received corticosteroid pharmacotherapy recently may be at an elevated risk of severe or fatal anaphylaxis, and this group in particular may benefit from extra steroids during an anaphylactic attack. The present authors' practice is to give steroids in all instances of anaphylaxis. Where oral administration may be problematic, the intravenous route of administration provides a better solution [1].

The majority of cases in which antihistamine and steroid therapy are used are associated with total remission of symptoms once steroids have been gradually withdrawn. For the minority, though, H1 blockers will be required on a long-term basis [1].

For use in an outpatient setting, oral histamine blockers and steroids are appropriate, with only a short course given, e.g. 2 days. Whether this is actually of benefit has not been demonstrated in any study up to now, but theoretically it should help [1].

A practical choice of oral steroid is prednisolone, the optimal dose of which is still moot. In adults, dividing a total daily dose of 1 mg/kg body weight into two is likely to be sufficient. There is no need to reduce the dose unless steroids have been administered over prolonged periods [1].

The following are the typical dosage regimens that physicians recommend, albeit there is no firm proof of their benefit in the treatment of anaphylactic reactions in Accident and Emergency. Bearing this in mind, what follows is not a definite recommendation, nor does it constitute any gold standard. In particular, supportive evidence for the role of H2 blockade is notably lacking.

H1 blockade as follows [1]:

- Diphenhydramine (Benadryl)—Adults: 25 mg orally qds for 2–5 days; Paediatric dosage: 1 mg/kg orally qds for 2–5 days
- Hydroxyzine (Atarax)—Adults: 25 mg orally tds for 2–5 days; Paediatric dosage: 1 mg/kg orally tds for 2–5 days

  Corticosteroid dosage is as follows [1]:

- Prednisone—Adults: 20–80 mg orally od for 2–5 days; Paediatric dosage: 0.5–1 mg/kg orally od for 2–5 days
- There are a large number of other suitable steroid regimens that may be utilised.

  H2 blockade as follows [1]:

- Cimetidine—300 mg orally qds for 2–5 days; Its usage is not recommended in paediatric cases.

Cases of typical idiopathic anaphylaxis may be beneficially treated by daily H1 and H2 blocker treatment, and, somewhat rarely, daily administration of corticosteroids.

Diphenhydramine and hydroxyzine are the usual first-line treatments if a continuous histamine blockade is needed. Second-generation histamine blockers produce less sedation and are thus preferable. For adults, the choices include: fexofenadine (Allegra) at a dose of 180 mg daily, loratadine (Claritin) at a dose of 10 mg daily, cetirizine (Zyrtec) at a dose of 10 mg daily, desloratadine (Clarinex) at a dose of 5 mg daily, and levocetirizine (Xyzal) at a dose of 5 mg daily. None of these agents has specifically been investigated as an anti-anaphylactic. Some specialists recommend adding prn antihistamines depending on whether they are tolerated and with a view to controlling breakthrough symptoms [1].

8.2.4.3 Patient Education

Avoiding known triggers is key, especially for young patients with allergies to foodstuffs. It is important to consider how allergens may contaminate food and how ingredients may not be fully listed. A study examining children with an allergy to food who attended a specialist clinic reported that 59% carried an adrenaline auto-injector, but 71% claimed they carried it with them at all times. The main predictor of remembering to carry the auto-injector was having been fully briefed in its usage [43].

Individuals who are allergic to specific anti-microbials need to be provided with a list detailing alternatives. This can be shown to physicians who want to prescribe antibiotics to them. Patients with insect venom allergy also must know how to avoid the trigger. Advise sufferers to keep away from perfumes or perfumed toiletries, especially flower-scented ones, as these can draw Hymenoptera species. Brightly coloured clothing may also attract bees or other pollinator species. They should steer clear of hives and nests and not use equipment that may disturb a nest.

Anyone with an allergy to Hymenoptera stings and who must work outside needs to have an auto-injector with them at all times. They should also be informed about desensitisation therapy. After using the auto-injector, there are side effects they need to be aware of, and they should know to seek follow-up in the event of having used the device [1].

8.3   Prognosis

Anaphylaxis resulting in death is not common, but not unusual either. Less extreme forms of anaphylactic response are even more common. It has been found that between 500 and 1000 fatal anaphylactic reactions occur on a yearly basis in the USA. The death rate amongst those known to have anaphylaxis is between 0.65 and 2% [44, 45].

Food allergy triggering anaphylaxis is the most common type outside clinical settings and has been calculated to cause 125 deaths annually in the USA. Severe reactions to penicillin happen in 1–5 individuals for every 10,000 courses of prescribed antibiotic. In the USA, Hymenoptera allergy officially causes possibly 100 fatal episodes annually although the true incidence may be higher [1].

In 1975, up to 900 deaths may have occurred as a result of anaphylactic reactions to radio-contrast media (RCM), some 0.009% of those exposed [46, 47]. According to one estimate, less osmotically active RCM agents account for 3.13% of mild to extreme reactions, whilst 12.66% of incidents are due to the ordinary RCM types. Treating prophylactically failed to reduce the incidence. Less osmotically active RCM also lowers the risk of fatal anaphylaxis to around 1 in 168,000 exposures [1, 48].

The principal mechanism leading to death in anaphylaxis is circulatory or respiratory arrest. One study looked at 214 deaths due to anaphylaxis and found 98 were produced by asphyxia (49 cases due to lower airway compromise [bronchospasm], 26 both upper and lower airways, and 23 upper airways only [angioedema]). Deaths resulting from acute spasm of the bronchi were confined to individuals who were already suffering from asthma [1].

References

1. Mustafa SS. Anaphylaxis. In: Kaliner MA, editor. Medscape. http://emedicine.medscape.com/article/135065-overview#showall. Accessed 14 July 2016.
2. Lieberman P. Anaphylaxis. In: Adkinson Jr NF, Bochner BS, Busse WW, Holgate ST, Lemanske Jr RF, Simons FER, editors. Middleton's allergy: principles and practice. 7th ed. Philadelphia, PA: Elsevier; 2009. p. 1027–49.
3. Lieberman P, Nicklas RA, Oppenheimer J, et al. The diagnosis and management of anaphylaxis practice parameter: 2010 update. J Allergy Clin Immunol. 2010;126(3):477–80.e1–42.
4. Lieberman P. Use of epinephrine in the treatment of anaphylaxis. Curr Opin Allergy Clin Immunol. 2003;3(4):313–8.
5. Sampson HA, Muñoz-Furlong A, Campbell RL, et al. Second symposium on the definition and management of anaphylaxis: summary report—second National Institute of Allergy and Infectious Disease/Food Allergy and Anaphylaxis Network symposium. Ann Emerg Med. 2006;47(4):373–80.
6. Kemp SF, Lockey RF, Simons FE. Epinephrine: the drug of choice for anaphylaxis. A statement of the World Allergy Organization. Allergy. 2008;63(8):1061–70.
7. Campbell RL. Anaphylaxis: emergency treatment. In: Walls RM, Feldweg AM, editors. Up to Date. http://www.uptodate.com/contents/anaphylaxis-emergency-treatment. Accessed 14 July 2016.
8. Lieberman P, Nicklas RA, Randolph C, et al. Anaphylaxis—a practice parameter update 2015. Ann Allergy Asthma Immunol. 2015;115:341.
9. Simons FE, Ardusso LR, Bilò MB, et al. World Allergy Organization anaphylaxis guidelines: summary. J Allergy Clin Immunol. 2011;127:587.
10. Soar J, Pumphrey R, Cant A, et al. Emergency treatment of anaphylactic reactions—guidelines for healthcare providers. Resuscitation. 2008;77:157.
11. Brown SG, Mullins RJ, Gold MS. Anaphylaxis: diagnosis and management. Med J Aust. 2006;185:283.

12. Muraro A, Roberts G, Clark A, et al. The management of anaphylaxis in childhood: position paper of the European academy of allergology and clinical immunology. Allergy. 2007;62:857.
13. Campbell RL, Li JT, Nicklas RA, et al. Emergency department diagnosis and treatment of anaphylaxis: a practice parameter. Ann Allergy Asthma Immunol. 2014;113:599.
14. Simons KJ, Simons FE. Epinephrine and its use in anaphylaxis: current issues. Curr Opin Allergy Clin Immunol. 2010;10:354.
15. Brown SG, Blackman KE, Stenlake V, Heddle RJ. Insect sting anaphylaxis; prospective evaluation of treatment with intravenous adrenaline and volume resuscitation. Emerg Med J. 2004;21:149.
16. Simons FE. First-aid treatment of anaphylaxis to food: focus on epinephrine. J Allergy Clin Immunol. 2004;113:837.
17. Simons FE, Gu X, Simons KJ. Epinephrine absorption in adults: intramuscular versus subcutaneous injection. J Allergy Clin Immunol. 2001;108:871.
18. Simons FE, Roberts JR, Gu X, Simons KJ. Epinephrine absorption in children with a history of anaphylaxis. J Allergy Clin Immunol. 1998;101:33.
19. Pumphrey RS. Fatal posture in anaphylactic shock. J Allergy Clin Immunol. 2003;112:451.
20. Brown SG. The pathophysiology of shock in anaphylaxis. Immunol Allergy Clin N Am. 2007;27:165.
21. Brown SG. Anaphylaxis: clinical concepts and research priorities. Emerg Med Australas. 2006;18:155.
22. Geerts BF, van den Bergh L, Stijnen T, et al. Comprehensive review: is it better to use the Trendelenburg position or passive leg raising for the initial treatment of hypovolemia? J Clin Anesth. 2012;24:668.
23. Simons FE. Anaphylaxis, killer allergy: long-term management in the community. J Allergy Clin Immunol. 2006;117:367.
24. Vadas P, Perelman B. Effect of epinephrine on platelet-activating factor-stimulated human vascular smooth muscle cells. J Allergy Clin Immunol. 2012;129:1329.
25. McLean-Tooke AP, Bethune CA, Fay AC, Spickett GP. Adrenaline in the treatment of anaphylaxis: what is the evidence? BMJ. 2003;327:1332.
26. Simons FE. Pharmacologic treatment of anaphylaxis: can the evidence base be strengthened? Curr Opin Allergy Clin Immunol. 2010;10:384.
27. Kemp SF, Lockey RF, Simons FE, World Allergy Organization ad hoc Committee on Epinephrine in Anaphylaxis. Epinephrine: the drug of choice for anaphylaxis. A statement of the World Allergy Organization. Allergy. 2008;63:1061.

28. Kounis NG. Coronary hypersensitivity disorder: the Kounis syndrome. Clin Ther. 2013;35:563.

29. Kanwar M, Irvin CB, Frank JJ, et al. Confusion about epinephrine dosing leading to iatrogenic overdose: a life-threatening problem with a potential solution. Ann Emerg Med. 2010;55:341.

30. Campbell RL, Bellolio MF, Knutson BD, et al. Epinephrine in anaphylaxis: higher risk of cardiovascular complications and overdose after administration of intravenous bolus epinephrine compared with intramuscular epinephrine. J Allergy Clin Immunol Pract. 2015;3:76.

31. Kmietowicz Z. UK trainee doctors are still unsure about how to treat anaphylaxis. BMJ. 2015;350:h171.

32. Halbrich M, Mack DP, Carr S, et al. CSACI position statement: epinephrine auto-injectors and children < 15 kg. Allergy Asthma Clin Immunol. 2015;11:20.

33. Sicherer SH, Simons FE, Section on Allergy and Immunology, American Academy of Pediatrics. Self-injectable epinephrine for first-aid management of anaphylaxis. Pediatrics. 2007;119:638.

34. Simons FE, Ardusso LR, Bilo MB, Cardona V, Ebisawa M, El-Gamal YM, et al. International consensus on (ICON) anaphylaxis. World Allergy Organ J. 2014;7(1):9. https://doi.org/10.1186/1939-4551-7-9.

35. Muraro A, Werfel T, Hoffmann-Sommergruber K, Roberts G, Beyer K, Bindslev-Jensen C, et al. EAACI food allergy and anaphylaxis guidelines: diagnosis and management of food allergy. Allergy. 2014;69(8):1008–25. https://doi.org/10.1111/all.12429.

36. Pharma D. EpiPen®/EpiPen® Jr. Prescribing Information 2012. 2014. https://www.epipen.ca/sites/default/files/pdf/.

37. SanofiAventis US. Auvi-Q prescribing information. Bridgewater, NJ: SanofiAventis US; 2012.

38. Canada S-A. Allerject® 0.15 mg/Allerject® 0.30 mg prescribing. Information. 2013;15:2014.

39. Dreborg S, Wen X, Kim L, Tsai G, Nevis I, Potts R, Chiu J, Dominic A, Kim H. Do epinephrine auto-injectors have an unsuitable needle length in children and adolescents at risk for anaphylaxis from food allergy? Allergy Asthma Clin Immunol. 2016;12:11. https://doi.org/10.1186/s13223-016-0110-8. eCollection 2016.

40. Wheeler DW, Carter JJ, Murray LJ, et al. The effect of drug concentration expression on epinephrine dosing errors: a randomized trial. Ann Intern Med. 2008;148:11.

41. Sheikh A, Ten Broek V, Brown SG, Simons FE. H1-antihistamines for the treatment of anaphylaxis: Cochrane systematic review. Allergy. 2007;62(8):830–7.

42. Choo KJ, Simons E, Sheikh A. Glucocorticoids for the treatment of anaphylaxis: Cochrane systematic review. Allergy. 2010;65(10):1205–11.
43. Demuth KA, Fitzpatrick AM. Epinephrine autoinjector availability among children with food allergy. Allergy Asthma Proc. 2011;32(4):295–300.
44. Bock SA, Muñoz-Furlong A, Sampson HA. Fatalities due to anaphylactic reactions to foods. J Allergy Clin Immunol. 2001;107(1):191–3.
45. Greenberger PA, Rotskoff BD, Lifschultz B. Fatal anaphylaxis: postmortem findings and associated comorbid diseases. Ann Allergy Asthma Immunol. 2007;98(3):252–7.
46. Shehadi WH. Adverse reactions to intravascularly administered contrast media. A comprehensive study based on a prospective survey. Am J Roentgenol Radium Therapy, Nucl Med. 1975;124(1):145–52.
47. Katayama H, Yamaguchi K, Kozuka T, Takashima T, Seez P, Matsuura K. Adverse reactions to ionic and nonionic contrast media. A report from the Japanese Committee on the Safety of Contrast Media. Radiology. 1990;175(3):621–8.
48. Greenberger PA, Patterson R. The prevention of immediate generalized reactions to radiocontrast media in high-risk patients. J Allergy Clin Immunol. 1991;87(4):867–72.

Chapter 9
Communication Strategies with Anaphylactic Patients and Their Families

9.1 Introduction: Communication Strategies with Anaphylactic Patients and Their Families

Allergies come in sixth place amongst the many chronic disorders which afflict Americans, and the annual cost for the more than 50 million individuals affected exceeds $18bn [1].

An exaggerated response to an otherwise innocuous substance by the immune system is the core concept of allergy. Such triggering substances are termed allergens. They may cause allergic patients to sneeze, cough, or experience pruritus. The spectrum of allergic responses extends from the mildly irritant to the potentially fatal. An allergic response may occur periodically, as occurs in hay fever, or may be more persistent, as happens with sinusitis or asthma [1].

Whilst it is typically not feasible to prevent an allergy *per se*, the occurrence of allergic reactions can be avoided. As soon as the allergic specificity is established, avoidance of the trigger can be undertaken. Some ways to achieve avoidance include remaining indoors with air conditioning active whilst the seasonal allergen abounds, keeping clear of specific foodstuffs and having a home environment free of dust mites and animal dander.

© Springer Nature Switzerland AG 2020
C. Cingi, N. B. Muluk, *Quick Guide to Anaphylaxis*,
https://doi.org/10.1007/978-3-030-33639-4_9

Symptom severity may also be adjusted by drugs which impede the allergic response or diminish symptoms, or injections may be used to provide immunisation against the response [1].

The highest severity of allergic response occurs with anaphylaxis. Symptoms of flushing, paraesthesia of the extremities or lips, feeling lightheaded and experiencing crushing sternal pressure may occur. Unless therapy is given, the patient may progress onto convulsions, cardiac rhythmic abnormalities, circulatory collapse, and compromised breathing. Anaphylaxis may be fatal. Triggers to anaphylaxis include foodstuffs, rubber, insect venom, and medication [1].

Those aspects of concordance with pharmacological treatment that are amenable to measurement, such as when treatment starts, what form it takes, and whether the patient perseveres or not, are all subject in varying ways to a matrix of interdependent factors: patient choice, perspective on therapy, personal needs, understanding sufficiently what the disease involves, the health risks they are aware of, economic factors, general healthcare knowledge, the patient's worries about prognosis, what the patient anticipates will occur with therapy, and anxiety about the likelihood of adverse events associated with various drugs [2].

9.2   Stress and Allergic Diseases

Whilst the ideal treatment would involve lowering stress levels or avoiding stress altogether, such a situation is seldom feasible within the framework of modern lifestyles. Thus, an approach utilising psychological techniques, physiological interventions, or medication, or a mixture of these, offers the best chance to provide patients with resilience to stress and with ways to manage stress effectively to enhance clinical outcomes [3, 4].

Multiple studies have demonstrated that psychological methods offer benefit in the prognosis for allergic disorders. Smyth et al. proved that writing therapy focusing on stressful life events can lead to improvement in symptomatology for asthmatic patients. Both biofeedback and imagination-based techniques provide benefit in managing asthma [5–7]. Huntley et al. [8] undertook a systematic review, which concluded that relaxation techniques improved outcomes in asthma, and psychotherapy has also been shown [9] to lessen asthma attack frequency in depressed patients and to reduce presentations at Accident and Emergency departments. Whilst there is evidence pointing towards the benefits in such treatments working through an adjusted Th1/Th2 balance, there is a need for further investigation before it can be confidently claimed that the psychological techniques assert a direct effect on clinical outcomes via immunological parameters [3].

Techniques that utilise physiological methods to manage allergic disorders encompass exercise regimes as well as non-allopathic medical modalities such as acupuncture, chiropraxy, and applied kinesiology. Possibly all such interventions exert their effects through lowering the allergy sufferer's stress level. Up to now, no study of robust methodological design has been able to demonstrate an unequivocal benefit from non-allopathic interventions, potentially due to the fact that the placebo effect is very marked in such studies and leads, via a psychophysiological effect on the immune system, to a decrease in allergic responses [10]. Exercise has been shown to produce differing effects on the immune system, depending on how severe the immune abnormality was initially. Children whose asthma is in the mild to moderate range can tolerate exercise-based programmes well and show improvements in both aerobic and anaerobic fitness afterwards [11]. For patients whose asthma is mild, exercise-based intervention led to better aerobic fitness, expanded ventilatory capacity, and a reduction in hyperpnoea [12]. Notwithstanding the benefit in such cases, it is noteworthy that patients whose asthma is inadequately controlled may actually deteriorate if subjected to high levels of exercise [3].

9.3 Social Communication Problems in Allergic Rhinitis

The ability to communicate effectively requires prior learning. Whilst almost all humans have an innate capacity to learn to speak, communicating well depends on taking the time to work on communicative competency. The process of communication is, in reality, somewhat complicated. One way of defining communication is as "the act of giving, receiving or exchanging information, ideas and opinions so that the message is completely understood by both parties" [13].

For certain disorders, the assessment of feelings of shame needs to depend on non-verbal clues. Shame may have negative consequences, such as failing to report aspects of symptomatology (whether physical or psychological), or resulting in disrupted communication within couples [14].

Cases of allergic rhinitis (AR) are typically associated with impaired activity levels and a reduced degree of social interaction. AR is a significant social issue. Morbidity associated with AR encompasses not merely physical or social function, but also related comorbidities and financial burdens [15].

In addition to the core AR symptoms of a blocked nose and rhinorrhoea, individuals with AR also report tiredness (46%), difficulty concentrating (32%), and lower productivity (23%) [16]. For AR patients who vary their dosage regime for OTC and prescribed drugs to adjust for ineffectiveness or reduced efficacy, the fact that such regimes do not provide relief all around the clock or have associated adverse effects meant higher expenditure and more issues for the patient [15]. AR was periodic in 64% of cases and chronic in the remaining 36%, with the chronic variant being the more bothersome type. Some 49% of cases where AR was of mild severity or periodic were over-medicated, whilst for cases of moderate to marked severity, 30% of the time the treatment was actually inadequate [17].

AR has effects on sufferers' mood, with many feeling exhausted, bad-tempered, and embarrassed [15]. Mood disorders and AR may also influence each other [18]. Associations between AR and feeling anxious, having depressed mood and even committing suicide have been described in the literature [19].

AR has a deleterious effect on social communicative abilities. Disruption to sleep and rhinorrhoea may lead to occupational problems as well as a deterioration in the life quality of sufferers. Occupational under-performance adds to the cost of AR itself. However, timely intervention in the form of supplying knowledge about AR and adroit treatment do lead to decreases in symptoms related to rhinorrhoea, sneeze, headache, and sleep disturbance. Such interventions therefore address the social isolation which AR may produce [13].

9.4 Communication Problems in Accident and Emergency (A + E) Departments

Communication issues are entwined with the processes and procedures employed by A + E. A + E care is generally multidisciplinary and involves a large number of different practitioners, hence information about diagnosis, past medical history, and treatment needs to be swiftly transferred between professionals. Given that it is usual for A + E doctors to consult the patient without the benefit of previous documentation, the records produced within A + E have a key role to play. Two main problem areas in information flow were noted by one study: medical records that were incomplete or that contained inconsistent information; and failures within the system of triage and handover. Both these problem areas had a negative effect on the safety of patients and decreased contentment with clinical outcomes within A + E [20].

It is vital that healthcare practitioners appreciate patients' illnesses and their past medical history in sufficient depth to enable treatment to be of high quality, even more so when acute services are being accessed. Despite this need, healthcare practitioners frequently felt the patient record was overly brief, condensed, and hard to decipher. Inadequacies of this kind could lead to misunderstanding, failure to act, or inappropriate emendations. Beyond this, the notes may be too fragmentary to permit triage or handover to happen [20].

Whilst handovers were considered adequate by some practitioners, many practitioners were able to provide concrete examples of where communication in a patient handover was insufficient or self-contradictory. One study uncovered a lack of standardisation in the way handover was performed, with such handover as does occur being verbal, written, structured, or casual, and sometimes being absent altogether [20].

Interpersonal communicative ability relates to how well doctors can communicate with patients or other doctors. A paper discussing interpersonal communication within an A + E setting examined the importance doctors attach to building rapport with the patient and showing empathy, alongside an evaluation of how doctors felt their abilities in this respect were inadequate, despite such skills being part of healthcare [20].

Only where practitioners have built a relationship on the basis of efficacy and respect can medicine produce high quality outcomes. A key aim in establishing such a relationship is to facilitate a safe and high quality healthcare experience for the patient [21–23].

Despite the fact that communication between doctors themselves and between doctors and nurses is a key element on how patient information accompanies the patient within A + E, the roles practitioners play may become blurred, with the potential for both professionals and patients to misunderstand or miscommunicate. Nurses might, for instance, be left to "cover" for a medical colleague, but with insufficient information to allow this to occur. Doctors may make the assumption that nurses have supplied key information to patients, whereas this information has not yet been given. Due to the patchiness associated with such a flow of information, nurses may lack the necessary resources to answer patients' concerns, and doctors may be in the dark about how well the patient appreciates the clinical situation, with the result that the patient's safety may be compromised and patients left dissatisfied [20].

9.4.1 Discrepancy Between Information Given to Doctors and Nurses

Nurses often experience being accosted by patients, who expect the nurse to be able to readily answer their healthcare questions. Since, however, nurses might not have read the full record, they may have an incomplete understanding of the situation. In this way, division of responsibility between doctors and nurses may impede the flow of information. One study records a practitioner's view of the A + E department as resembling a factory, both physically and symbolically [20].

Whilst there is a general consensus amongst both doctors and nurses that empathic relationships that are conducive to rapport are key to treating patients, many professionals stress safety as their key priority, thereby indicating that they fail to link the two concepts in their mind [20]. Such a separation is in stark contrast to contemporary views on patient-centred healthcare, which stress that the communicating of clinical information and the establishment of rapport proceed hand-in-hand. Indeed, Slade et al. [4] have persuasively argued that communication and rapport building should happen together and that to "deliver care effectively, clinicians must communicate care effectively" [24].

9.4.2 Lack of Focus on Empathy and Rapport

Empathy has been conceptualised by Brock and Salinsky [25] as "the skills used to decipher and respond to the thoughts and feelings passing from the patient to the physician". Leach [26] saw rapport as a kind of "therapeutic alliance" built by doctors and patients, the basis for which is a shared understanding of how the patient sees the situation, and involving mutual trust and working together. An empirical study noted significant synchrony between cardiac rates of clinicians and patients engaged in psychotherapy and indicating that rapport had been established [27].

Slade et al. [21] revealed much to support the notion that the way a doctor establishes and bolsters the interpersonal relationship affects how effectively doctors and patients can communicate with each other. To put it another way, rapport building and empathy, far from being additional tasks for the practitioner, are the keystone in effective communication within a healthcare setting.

9.5   Communicating with and Caring for Patients and Their Families Following an Anaphylactic Episode

Once an anaphylactic reaction has taken place, tailored information may play a role in stopping recurrence or mitigating the severity of future episodes. Where clinicians experience a sense that they lack the training to tailor such information, it may be helpful to involve an allergy specialist [28, 29]. On occasion, a patient will attend a consultation only long after the initial anaphylactic event, in which case the likely allergenic trigger may be obscured by the passage of time. The experience of an allergy specialist may help elucidate the likely causes. Patients may be willing to take part in allergy testing with the aim of isolating the particular allergen and thus being able to contemplate avoiding the allergen or undergoing specific immunotherapy [30–34].

Avoiding triggers is the key to preventing recurrence, but absolute avoidance may be impracticable, particularly if the allergen is a foodstuff or insect venom [30, 32, 35]. All individuals with a history of anaphylaxis need to be issued with a manufactured adrenaline auto-injector [29, 36]. Used appropriately, auto-injectors can prevent the progression of an anaphylactic reaction to an untreatable state [37]. Patients need to be aware of how to summon an ambulance or attend the closest A + E to undergo observation following administration of the auto-injector [29, 36]. Three makes of auto-injector marketed in the USA are Epipen®, Twinject®, and Adrenaclick®. It is imperative that both doctors and allergy sufferers know how to administer the device. In a number of retrospective studies looking at auto-injector use, even when auto-injectors were used inappropriately or injected at the wrong anatomical site, invasive treatment was seldom deemed necessary and associated adverse effects were of brief duration.

Acknowledgements We would like to express our gratitude to Associate Professor Can Cemal Cingi, for his contribution to this chapter on this specialized aspect of communication.

References

1. Allergies. Centers for Disease Control and Prevention. https://www.cdc.gov/healthcommunication/toolstemplates/entertainmented/tips/Allergies.html. Accessed 6 June 2019.
2. Calderon MA, Cox L, Casale TB, Mösges R, Pfaar O, Malling HJ, Sastre J, Khaitov M, Demoly P. The effect of a new communication template on anticipated willingness to initiate or resume allergen immunotherapy: an internet-based patient survey. Allergy Asthma Clin Immunol. 2015;11(1):17. https://doi.org/10.1186/s13223-015-0083-z. eCollection 2015.
3. Dave ND, Xiang L, Rehm KE, Marshall GD Jr. Stress and allergic diseases. Immunol Allergy Clin N Am. 2011;31(1):55–68. https://doi.org/10.1016/j.iac.2010.09.009.
4. Barton C, Clarke D, Sulaiman N, Abramson M. Coping as a mediator of psychosocial impediments to optimal management and control of asthma. Respir Med. 2003;97(7):747–61.
5. Lehrer PM, Vaschillo E, Vaschillo B, et al. Biofeedback treatment for asthma. Chest. 2004;126(2):352–61.
6. Epstein GN, Halper JP, Barrett EA, et al. A pilot study of mind-body changes in adults with asthma who practice mental imagery. Altern Ther Health Med. 2004;10(4):66–71.
7. Freeman LW, Welton D. Effects of imagery, critical thinking, and asthma education on symptoms and mood state in adult asthma patients: a pilot study. J Altern Complement Med. 2005;11(1):57–68.
8. Huntley A, White AR, Ernst E. Relaxation therapies for asthma: a systematic review. Thorax. 2002;57(2):127–31.
9. Lehrer P, Feldman J, Giardino N, Song HS, Schmaling K. Psychological aspects of asthma. J Consult Clin Psychol. 2002;70(3):691–711.

10. Markham AW, Wilkinson JM. Complementary and alternative medicines (CAM) in the management of asthma: an examination of the evidence. J Asthma. 2004;41(2):131–9.

11. Counil FP, Varray A, Matecki S, et al. Training of aerobic and anaerobic fitness in children with asthma. J Pediatr. 2003;142(2):179–84.

12. Hallstrand TS, Bates PW, Schoene RB. Aerobic conditioning in mild asthma decreases the hyperpnea of exercise and improves exercise and ventilatory capacity. Chest. 2000;118(5):1460–9.

13. Cingi CC, Muluk NB, Hancı D, Şahin E. Impacts of allergic rhinitis in social communication, quality of life and behaviours of the patients. Allergy Disord Ther. 2015;2:002.

14. Ekman P, Rosenberg E. What the face reveals: basic and applied studies of spontaneous expression using the Facial Action Coding System (FACS). New York: Oxford University Press; 2005.

15. Nathan RA. The burden of allergic rhinitis. Allergy Asthma Proc. 2007;28:3–9.

16. Keith PK, Desrosiers M, Laister T, Schellenberg RR, Waserman S. The burden of Allergic Rhinitis (AR) in Canada: perspectives of physicians and patients. Allergy Asthma Clin Immunol. 2012;8:7.

17. Van Hoecke H, Vastesaeger N, Dewulf L, Sys L, van Cauwenberge P. Classification and management of allergic rhinitis patients in general practice during pollen season. Allergy. 2006;61:705–11.

18. Sansone RA, Sansone LA. Allergic rhinitis: relationships with anxiety and mood syndromes. Innov Clin Neurosci. 2011;8:12–7.

19. Postolache TT, Komarow H, Tonelli LH. Allergy: a risk factor for suicide? Curr Treat Options Neurol. 2008;10:363–76.

20. Pun JK, Matthiessen CM, Murray KA, Slade D. Factors affecting communication in emergency departments: doctors and nurses' perceptions of communication in a trilingual ED in Hong Kong. Int J Emerg Med. 2015;8(1):48. https://doi.org/10.1186/s12245-015-0095-y. Epub 2015 Dec 15.

21. Slade D, Manidis M, McGregor J, Scheeres H, Stein-Parbury J, Dunston R, et al. Communicating in hospital emergency departments: final report. Sydney: University of Technology Sydney; 2011. p. 2011.

22. Little P, Everitt H, Williamson I, Warner G, Moore M, Gould C, et al. Observational study of effect of patient centredness and positive approach on outcomes of general practice consultations. BMJ. 2001;323:908–11. https://doi.org/10.1136/bmj.323.7318.908.

23. Williams S, Weinman J, Dale J. Doctor-patient communication and patient satisfaction: a review. Fam Pract. 1998;15(5):480–92. https://doi.org/10.1093/fampra/15.5.480.

24. Slade D, Chandler E, Pun J, Lam M, Matthiessen CMIM, William G, et al. Effective healthcare worker-patient communication in Hong Kong accident and emergency departments. Hong Kong J Emerg Med. 2015;22:69–83.

25. Brock C, Salinsky J. Empathy: an essential skill for understanding the physician-patient relationship. Fam Med. 1993;25:245–8.
26. Leach J. Rapport: a key to treatment success. Complement Ther Clin Pract. 2005;11(4):262–5. https://doi.org/10.1016/j.ctcp.2005.05.005.
27. Levenson RW, Ruef AM. Physiological aspects of emotional knowledge and rapport. In: Ickes W, editor. Empathic accuracy. New York: Guilford; 1997. p. 44–72.
28. Kemp SF, Lockey RF, Simons FE. Epinephrine: the drug of choice for ananphylaxis. A statement of the World Allergy Organization. Allergy. 2008;63(8):1061–70.
29. Oswalt ML, Kemp SF. Anaphylaxis: office management and prevention. Immunol Allergy Clin N Am. 2007;27(2):177–91.
30. Joint Task Force on Practice Parameters; American Academy of Allergy, Asthma and Immunology; American College of Allergy, Asthma, and Immunology; Joint Council on Allergy, Asthma and Immunology. The diagnosis and management of anaphylaxis: an updated practice parameter (published correction appears in J Allergy Clin Immunol. 2008;122(1):68). J Allergy Clin Immunol. 2005;115(3 suppl 2):S483–523.
31. Arnold JJ, Williams PM. Anaphylaxis: recognition and management. Am Fam Physician. 2011;84(10):1111–8.
32. Kemp SF. Navigating the updated anaphylaxis parameters. Allergy Asthma Clin Immunol. 2007;3(2):40–9.
33. Simons FE. Anaphylaxis (published correction appears in J Allergy Clin Immunol. 2010;126(4):885). J Allergy Clin Immunol. 2010;125(2 suppl 2):S161–81.
34. Ben-Shoshan M, Clark AE. Anaphylaxis: past, present and future. Allergy. 2011;66(1):1–14.
35. Sampson HA, Muñoz-Furlong A, Campbell RL, et al. Second symposium on the definition and management of anaphylaxis: summary report—second National Institute of Allergy and Infectious Disease/Food Allergy and Anaphylaxis Network Symposium. Ann Emerg Med. 2006;47(4):373–80.
36. Kemp SF. Office approach to anaphylaxis: sooner better than later. Am J Med. 2007;120(8):664–8.
37. Wheeler DW, Carter JJ, Murray LJ, et al. The effect of drug concentration expression on epinephrine dosing errors: a randomized trial. Ann Intern Med. 2008;148(1):11–4.

Printed in the United States
By Bookmasters